The IBS Breakthrough

FAIR WINDS
PRESS
GLOUCESTER, MASSACHUSETTS

The IBS
Breakthrough

Healing
Irritable Bowel Syndrome for Good
with Ancient
Chinese Medicine

LEIGH FORTSON
with Bing Lee, Dipl. Ac.

First published in the USA in 2001 by
Fair Winds Press
33 Commercial Street
Gloucester, MA   01930

10   9   8   7   6   5   4   3   2   1

Printed and bound in Canada

ISBN 1-931412-62-6

Cover design by Jane Ramsey
Book design by SYP Design & Production, Inc.

*The information in this book is for educational
purposes only. It is not intended to replace the
advice of a physician or medical practitioner.
Please see your health care provider before beginning any new health program.*

To Tucker and Lyric, the two most delicious morsels on earth.
And to Eddie, for keeping my heart a-throbbing.

ACKNOWLEDGMENTS

Many, many thanks to everyone who gave their stories, knowledge, and resources to make this book possible.

To Bing Lee: Thank you for keeping my body balanced and the laughter flowing. You're a hero to many, and my mentor and friend.

To Barbara Neighbors Deal: Who wouldn't die for an agent with the last name "Deal"? Of all you've done for me, I most appreciate your love and friendship, which I value to the depths.

To Holly Schmidt at Fair Winds Press: From tomatoes to the written word, I deeply appreciate what we share.

To the Grand Junction talent of Tomas E. Lynch, M.T.O.M.; Deborah Kinnes, Dipl. Ac., Dipl. C.H., C.M.T.; Kristin Dillon Lummis, supreme researcher; Dr. Louis DePalma, for insights and wisdom; and my friend Andrea, who listens.

Finally, to Dr. Alan Bensoussan; Barbara Mitchell at the Acupuncture Alliance (even during earthquake season!); Dr. Robert Yuan; Al Stone; Dr. Claire Cassidy; and Sheree Lane at *The Journal of Alternative and Complementary Medicine.*

TABLE OF CONTENTS

PREFACE

Joanne's Story, Age 38

I started having abdominal pains when I was about 16 years old. They seemed to get better when I went to the bathroom, but pretty soon I began having either diarrhea or constipation—both accompanied by cramps. The cramps could be incapacitating. Once, the pain was so bad that I collapsed. I was terrified that I had cancer or something life threatening, so I finally told my mother about it. She seemed embarrassed by the whole idea, but decided it was worth a trip to the doctor.

The doctor did a series of very painful tests on me and finally concluded that nothing was wrong. I figured it was just me, that I was somehow a freak or was being punished for something. Our family was religious, and I was taught that bad things happened when people did bad things. So, I began a life lived in pain and filled with overwhelming feelings of powerlessness and guilt. This was my own silent hell.

A few years passed like this, and I went to college. I was terrified of dorm life, where I would have to share a bathroom. The pain I suffered from was intense, and the alternating episodes of diarrhea and constipation became worse. I ended up paying a girl to switch dorm rooms with me because hers was right next to the bathroom. As time went on, I spent so much time in the bathroom that I could identify people by their shoes.

During classes, I always sat near the door so I could bolt to the toilet if the need arose. Just before the cramping started, I would break into a sweat. I felt so conspicuous, and I continued to believe that I was being singled out and punished for some horrible deed I had committed.

One day a friend asked why I always ran to the bathroom instead of walked. I confided in her and she said, "I've got that, too. There's nothing worse than a spastic colon."

It had a name! I couldn't believe it. I couldn't believe I wasn't the only one going through the agony and humiliation. My friend suggested I go back to a doctor and talk about what could be done for it. I went to the college medical clinic and they agreed that my condition was irritable bowel syndrome. The doctor suggested eating a high-fiber diet, taking over-the-counter laxatives for the constipation, and using Kaopectate to control the diarrhea. I didn't leave the house without them.

After a few years of relying on my "elixirs," my poor body was all messed up. Every symptom I suffered from got worse. I went to another doctor, who prescribed a powerful antacid. It didn't work. Even though my social life had improved, I felt like I was slowly disappearing. It seemed to me that my life was being lived in the bathroom.

Through the years, I've been given countless drugs. I've endured side effect after side effect, including horrible fatigue, no sex drive, hives, insomnia, and dry mouth. I know every bathroom on the way to work, and I only eat at restaurants with multistall facilities. I have turned down more invitations to go to dinner than I have accepted. In some ways, I have become a bit of a recluse.

Ironically, I met a man while waiting in line at a public restroom. We began to talk, and he took an interest in me. It was hard for me to allow him into my life because I was having a hard time dealing with my own problems—how could I expect him to understand? He persisted, though, and after listening to me and watching how I lived, he helped me accept that I wasn't helping myself. I had given up. Through his love and support, I've found the strength to keep looking for answers. Never in a million years did I think that waiting in line to go to the bathroom would introduce me to my motive for healing myself.

INTRODUCTION

It's not something you typically hear about at cocktail parties, especially if you don't attend them. And, if you're like a lot of people who suffer from irritable bowel syndrome (IBS), you might shy away from at least *some* social activities out of fear that you may have an "attack" while there. Indeed, life with IBS can feel like you've been hijacked by an invisible enemy who has the power to assault you, without warning, at any time of the day or night.

It's not something people tend to discuss at the dinner table, either. Or with friends, family, or even their doctors. Although a staggering 20 percent of America's population knows how debilitating IBS can be, many people refuse to tell family members or their health care professional that they experience it. After all, it's a deeply personal condition and it's relatively easy to hide. There is no physical deterioration—no ulcers, cancerous cells, atrophied muscles, bruises, or scars. Even medical tests reveal no physiological decline. Because of that—and sheer embarrassment—some people successfully deny for years that they have IBS. Until one day they're stricken with so much pain that they literally cannot move, or they have a nightmarish accident. That's when a doctor hears about it, very often from the worried spouse or parent of a reluctant and mortified patient.

Although you may not be comfortable discussing the subject, the truth is that poop happens—and there's no reason to be ashamed of it. As Taro Gomi puts it in her classic children's book *Everyone Poops*, "All living things eat, so everyone poops." In this book, we'll address *how* it happens and in what ways Chinese medicine can ensure that it happens without pain and with regularity. To do that, however, we're going to be candid and ignore the stigma associated with the condition.

Let's look for a moment at common attitudes regarding bathroom activities. For some reason, people who jump off the toilet having had glorious success at evacuation often enjoy announcing it to the entire world, probably because they feel so good. Their theme song might be "Wild Thing—I Think You Move Me!"

Meanwhile, those who have trouble in the *salle de bain* slink away, hoping to be and stay invisible. They may feel ashamed, embarrassed, damp with perspiration from the pain, weak from diarrhea, and anxious about an attack that may hit on the freeway, in a bus or subway, or even in an elevator. Their theme song (which is neither sung nor spoken) could be "Make the World Go Away."

Humiliation is as common a symptom of IBS as the urgent need to defecate. The real tragedy, however, is that feeling bad about yourself and hiding concerns from others—those who love you or who could help manage the inconveniences—may exacerbate the problem. And Western science can now document a premise that traditional Chinese medicine (TCM) has functioned on for hundreds of years: Our minds and bodies work together to create overall health and well-being. Because of this connection, shutting down, masking the pain, and denying it to others only adds psychological discomfort to a physical imbalance.

It makes sense that if you approach this condition openly, with a sense of adventure and a dash of humor (rather than with feelings of disgrace and pessimism), you will have greater success at easing both your physical and your psychological "dis-ease." You'll also be closer to altering your symptoms and pinpointing their causes, because you'll have a more objective view of what contributes to the dynamic and therefore a better understanding of what course to take to change it. And with the new perspective you'll gain on this condition, you're more likely to be open to the treatments we suggest.

Our first suggestion, then, is to relax about the subject matter itself. Surely it's no laughing matter, but having some humor about it helps. Humor may not be the only medicine, but we know that it helps in the healing process. In fact, there is now evidence that laughter increases the heart rate, deepens breathing, improves blood circulation, stimulates muscles, lowers blood pressure, reduces stress, aids in digestion, helps you sleep, and releases endorphins that reduce pain. Plus, it makes you more fun to be with.

For all those reasons, we're going to be a little goofy in places. Our intention with the tone of this book is to lighten your load (so to speak) and to help flush away the strain of shame and embarrassment that may shadow you. We're going to laugh at how absurd it is that those who are regular feel free to happily proclaim it, while many of those who aren't regular remain collectively mute—or verbally constipated.

For this book, at least, forget about formalities and inhibitions! We're going to talk about this condition frankly and with an occasional giggle. We'll introduce ideas on how TCM can help you change your theme to "Born Free!" or "Gotta Dance!" (Or whatever song liberates your spirits as well as your colon.) In essence, we just want to take the "shhhhhh" out of "it," and have a little fun in the process.

By the way: We won't be at all insulted if you leave this book in the bathroom, within arm's reach of the toilet. In fact, we encourage it because we're guaranteed you'll have plenty of opportunities to read it!

Michael's Story, Age 56

Back in the early 1970s, I worked as a pediatric respiratory therapist in a children's hospital in Cleveland, but I lived way out in the southeast suburbs.

It was about 11 p.m. and I had just gotten off an evening shift. It was the dead of winter in the Snow Belt, and it was snowing like crazy. I was about halfway home, slowly wending my way through the icy-slick and deserted streets, when I became aware of that sticky dryness in my mouth, and then a slight ringing in my ears. These are the subtle and unwelcome early warning signs that an attack of IBS was looming. I drove faster.

The icy streets, houses, telephone poles, and trees blurred into a world of bright white. Only the faint yellow lines beneath the ice were clear, and they pointed me in the direction of the comfort and warmth of my toilet. Then the gurgling began. Slowly at first, then rising like hot lentil soup in the pressure cooker of my gut. It was going to be The Big One.

"I'm not going to make it!" I thought. "Wait—the SOHIO Gas Station!"

Oh, the horror. The SOHIO's bathroom was unheated, and it was 20 below zero outside. The restroom was filthy and they never had toilet paper, but it didn't matter—it sounded better to me every second. The sweat began to bead on my brow, which was deeply furrowed by then. I peered into the whiteness of winter, looking, searching, desperate to find the SOHIO. Then I realized I had already passed it. It was behind me, two, maybe three miles. "I can do this!" I told myself, bracing for another few minutes.

Looking for a left-turn lane to make a U-turn, my world became a blurring, ever-tightening race against time. When suddenly, out of the whiteness, there was something red. Red! The lights of the SOHIO? I instinctively slammed my foot on the parking brake, and my totally trick '68 Olds 4-4-2 executed the perfect 180 born of forbidden experiences a boy can only have in places like Cleveland.

As the rear swung around, headlights flashing against the wall of snow, I completed a nearly faultless turn and launched into a flurry of spinning Tiger Paw tires back toward the salvation of the SOHIO. And then I saw it. In the rearview mirror. My eyes glazed over in sheer terror at the sight that all speeding IBSers dread: Blue lights alternating with red lights! "No! No! Not now! Why isn't he at the pancake house flirting with Bernice? I'll get ten points off my license and ten pounds of poop in my pants if the SOB pulls me over! He's pulling me over! Okay, think, think!"

As he walked up to the car, I could tell by my intestinal hourglass that I had no more than five minutes left before I exploded. I scanned the possible scenarios and tried to imagine what was more believable:

1. *"The hospital called me in . . . patient on a ventilator . . .
   dying . . . no one can save him but me. . . . See my white
   jacket and beeper? Ventilator is malfunctioning!"*
2. *"I have diarrhea really, really, really bad, officer. Really."*
   *(The term irritable bowel syndrome hadn't been invented yet,
   but everyone could relate to an attack of diarrhea, right?)*

Thoughts raced through my mind. Everyone who is caught
speeding says they have diarrhea, and no cop in Cleveland was
going to buy that from a kid pulling u-turns on Warrensville Road
in a 4-4-2 at 11:30 at night in a snowstorm! And if he didn't buy
it, then I would have to let loose in my car. My beautiful 4-4-2!
Black leather bucket seats and all! No way!

He came to the door and I immediately rolled down my win-
dow and frantically began the verbal babble: "I'm sorry, officer, but
I am on call! On call! See my beeper? Babies' and Children's
Hospital! Ventilator malfunction! Baby! Machine stopped! I gotta
get there, now!"

It looked like he was buying it. If he called the hospital, my
buddy on the night shift would cover for me. Oh—my—God, it looked
like it was working!

"Please! A life is in the balance!" I went on ad nauseum.

Cocking his head, he gave me that "I'm not sure" look, then he
flipped his book closed and turned away. I was clear!

I grabbed the key and turned over the ignition That car never
sounded so good as it did that moment. I rammed it into first gear
when the cop did a quick turn, looked at me, and said, pointing in
the opposite direction, "The hospital's that way!"

Oh, no! It was true, though: The hospital was north, and I was
running a two-ton, 400-horsepower luge south!

Feeling the pressure inching its way to freedom, the truth finally
came out of me like a tidal wave. The stress of the moment raised
the urgency so much that I did a peppermint twist in my seat to
keep things contained.

"Okay, okay, I've got diarrhea really bad and it's coming
really soon! Honest, officer, I am so sorry, but I was sick, I was in

the hospital, I had surgery. Please, please let me go to the SOHIO station up there and you can arrest me when I'm done! Or, where's the Warrensville police station? Does it have a bathroom? Which is closer? Please, I am not kidding! Please? Follow me. I don't care. Impound the car, just please let me go to the station or I'm going to do it right here in the road because I cannot stop this!"

With a heavy sigh, the man who had heard it all, standing in a snowstorm at 11:30 at night, was hearing it again.

"Okay, kid. But I am going with you and you are going to court for cutting that donut in the middle of the—hey, slow down!"

That was all he had to say. I was out of there, blowing snow and ice all over his galoshes, spinning, careening up the road to the red beacon of the SOHIO station.

Sliding into the parking lot, I threw the car in neutral, slammed on the parking brake, flung open the door, and flew—slipping and sliding—toward the motherly bosom of the sign that read "Men."

Upon arrival, the usual ritual began. I slammed open the stall door and slammed down the seat. I proceeded to conduct my ugly business in the rudest possible fashion with all manner of animal-istic sounds issuing forth from both ends of my body. I could only imagine what fate awaited me outside the half-closed door.

After what was probably only 30 minutes but what seemed an eternity of spasmodic, hideously painful interplay with the porce-lain god, my eyes settled on the space between the floor and the door. I sat watching the snowflakes drift in through the dried and broken seal, pondering my fate. The blue and red flashing lights continued to be visible under the door, reflected in the accumula-tion of snow. I shook my head and gathered myself up. I arduously cleaned myself with the meager materials provided by a rich oil company: a few paper towels and a frozen bar of Lava soap. I still remember the unwelcome sensation of the "cleansing volcanic pumice."

My urgent task finally complete, I turned to the door, ready to face my fate. I opened the door slowly, peering into the white night, only to stop in my tracks. He was gone! I stood in the door, *squinting into the falling snow to see if he was anywhere near. He wasn't. Half-amazed, half-terrified that he would return with a brigade of generals, I walked gingerly to my car. I got in, closed the door, and rubbed my hands together for warmth. He still wasn't there. I decided it was safe to leave. I shifted into first gear, looked up, and there before me, written on my windshield in bold letters justly lightly snowed-over, it read:*

I BELIEVE YOU.

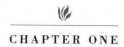

CHAPTER ONE

Recognizing and Identifying IBS

I was 14 years old when I had my first attack. It was summertime, and I was visiting my grandparents in Connecticut. They had arranged for my cousin to take me out for a ride in her sailboat, although I'm a mountain-girl, prone to motion sickness, and have always been slightly afraid of water. I went anyway, although I would have preferred a visit to my dentist.

We rocked farther and farther out to sea in what seemed like the tiniest, scariest, most unsteady marine craft ever made. I kept looking at the shore, wishing we could turn back but knowing it would be rude to ask. My cousin's passion was sailing. She was known throughout the eastern seaboard for winning races and successfully passing on her skills to eager wanna-be sailors. I was supposed to be privileged to get a ride with her, but instead I was terrified, feeling woozy, and longing for the mountainous West and Mom—both of which were thousands of miles away.

Then it struck: a pain so sharp, so deep in my gut that I thought I had been stabbed. I froze with the pain. Although I was barely able to move, I instinctively reached down and held my stomach. My breath stopped. I was overtaken by the pain, wracked by it. I had never felt anything so extreme in my life. A drop of perspiration fell from my temple, and for a fleeting moment I thought was going to die on the horrible waters of Long Island Sound in the company of my cousin, with whom I had nothing in common.

Then I heard a voice inside my head say, "Breathe. Just breathe." I did, but I must have let out an unconscious moan. My cousin, whose hard gaze had been set on her course, turned my way. Upon looking at me, she asked matter-of-factly, "You gonna puke?"

"I might," I grunted. It was my only out. Rolling her eyes and shaking her head at my landlubber ways, she jerked the boat back in the direction of the shore.

My grandparents were waiting with eager smiles, but they were confused about why we were returning so soon. Before I could say anything—I was uncertain whether I could stand upright with the excruciating pain that still twisted my guts—my cousin said, "Couldn't handle it. She's sick."

My grandmother had been a nurse in her earlier years, and she came quickly to my side. I must have been an appropriate shade of green because no one doubted that I was experiencing just another case of seasickness. When I tried to stand, however, the wrenching pain doubled me over, and my grandmother sensed something more. "Are you okay? What's wrong?"

With as much dignity as I could muster, I whispered, "I need to go to the bathroom."

My cousin snickered, while my grandfather looked concerned. My grandmother escorted me to the outdoor beach stalls, and I closed the door, hoping she would join the others on the dock so I could privately talk myself out of this pain. But instead she stood at the door, waiting for a report and hoping I would vomit to relieve the symptoms she believed the choppy waters had imposed upon me. The urge I had was not to vomit, though, but to defecate. Bent over in agony, I sat upon the porcelain throne, fighting off the spasms of pain that kept everything locked up tight in my gut. I was dripping with sweat and mortified to be the center of attention in the middle of a family vacation. And I was wondering, somewhere deep within, if something was indeed terribly, terribly wrong with me.

After about ten minutes on the toilet—having produced nothing—the pain began to subside. By then, my grandmother knew that the problem was in my abdomen, and she promised to feed me some prunes when we got back to her house. I acted as normally as possible, even though I wanted to crawl beneath the sand and never be seen again. I was completely spent. My knees wobbled as I walked. My cousin smirked. My grandfather looked alarmed upon seeing me, and he warmly took me into his arms. "Let's go home," he whispered. My eyes welled up with tears and I nodded.

I haven't set foot in a sailboat since.

> "Treasure the love you receive above all. It will survive long after your good health has vanished."
>
> —Og Mandino

Defining IBS

As was true in my case, the first bout with irritable bowel syndrome (IBS) can cause sheer panic. The pain is sudden, severe, and shocking. If it occurs in a public place, it can be horrifying. If there isn't a bathroom nearby to answer to the desperate physical call, it's paralyzing. You can't help wondering, "What will happen if I can't hold it in?" Suddenly, all feelings of control are replaced with vulnerability and terror. The bottom line: It's no picnic.

In broad terms, there are two types of IBS: the painful, cramping symptoms associated with a spastic colon, and painless—but chronic—diarrhea. As severe and debilitating as it can be, IBS is considered a *functional disorder* because there are no signs of disease when the colon is examined. It has no relationship to, nor does it rank among, the more serious gastrointestinal conditions such as Crohn's disease, an inflamed stomach or pancreas, colon cancer, lupus, an imbalance of stomach acids, ulcers, scleroderma, or the inflammatory bowel disease found in ulcerative colitis. It also does not cause colon or rectal cancer, require surgery, or shorten or threaten a person's life (even though it's reasonable to think that it could). In fact, most people experience fewer symptoms of the condition as they age. Some are even symptom-free by midlife.

Even so, IBS is the most common gastrointestinal disorder for which people visit a health care professional. The International Foundation for Bowel Dysfunction (imagine the jokes that circulate around those offices) claims that the disorder is second only to the common cold as a cause of absenteeism from work or school. That's synonymous with 3 million physician visits per year, costing upwards of $8 million. Even though cases range from mild to extreme, the people who live with IBS agree that it is, at least, life altering.

> "There are only two reasons to sit in the back of an airplane: Either you have diarrhea or you're anxious to meet people who do."
> —Henry Kissinger

Also known as a spastic colon, irritable colon syndrome, and mucous colitis, symptoms of IBS typically show up for the first time during adolescence or young adulthood. Still, people of all ages and races, in all countries, and of all socioeconomic circles experience it. Worldwide, twice as many women as men have it, although many professionals believe this simply reflects that more women than men visit doctors and therefore more women than men have been diagnosed. Most health care providers believe there are far more people who live with the condition than are accounted for because the majority of people *don't* seek help.

Dr. Rona Levy of the University of Washington conducted a study revealing that patients with IBS were slightly more likely to have children who would develop the condition. It's not known if this is due to genetics, socialization, family dynamics, or learned health care behavior. In another study, Dr. Arnold Wald of the University of Pittsburgh Medical Center found a high prevalence of anxiety disorder—particularly panic disorder, mood disorder, and somatization disorder—among patients with IBS. Dr. Wald emphasized, however, that IBS itself is not a psychological disorder.

> "For every experience in the mind, there is a corresponding change in the physiology of our body. We have a vast internal pharmacy that can be accessed through conscious choices we make in our lives. A key tenet of mind-body medicine is that health is not the mere absence of disease. Rather, it is the dynamic integration of our environment, body, mind and spirit."
>
> —Deepak Chopra
> *Namaste* online newsletter

Diagnosis: Two Approaches

In traditional Chinese medicine (TCM), recognizing and acting on what is unique about each individual is key to both diagnosing and treating any imbalance. Everyone has a unique physiological, psychological, and spiritual system that the doctor considers. The doctor may ask questions and look for clues that you don't think are relevant to your situation, but TCM looks at the big picture, the whole self, since the philosophy is rooted in a belief that all things are related. The overall objective of TCM is to ascertain the *relationship of all contributing parts* of the dysfunction and to assist in reestablishing the balance that leads to good health and well-being.

Historically, Western medicine has taken a narrower approach. It looks at parts of the picture and typically treats symptoms, rather than identifying causes or the relationships between the parts. As such, a diagnosis of IBS is based on a list of mostly physical symptoms. In the next section, we will present Western medicine's definition and diagnosis of IBS; later in the book, we will help you recognize and identify what is unique about your own interrelated physiology, psychology, environment, and sense of purpose. This will enable you to look at the bigger picture and understand the more abstract contributions to the disorder. For those new to alternative medicine or TCM, learning to look outside

Western medicine's allopathic "box" takes time and trust. We'll ease into it so you can integrate the information in as useful a way as possible.

The Western View of IBS

To determine if you have IBS, most medical doctors would probably turn to a standard diagnostic system called the Rome criteria. According to that standard, you must have experienced typical symptoms—such as abdominal pain with diarrhea, constipation, or both—for at least three months prior to your visit. Additionally, according to the Mayo Foundation for Medical Education, you need to have experienced at least two of the four conditions below for at least 25 percent of the three months prior:

- A change in the frequency or consistency of your stool (For example, you may change from having one normal, formed stool every day to several loose stools. Or, you may have only one hard stool every three or four days.)
- Straining, urgency, or a feeling that you can't empty your bowels completely
- Mucus in your stool
- Bloating or a feeling of abdominal distension

Although not included in the Rome criteria, other common symptoms include:

- Sudden, urgent need to use the toilet
- Painful gas (upon passing gas, pain usually ceases)
- Nausea
- Heavy perspiration
- Feelings of fullness or lack of appetite
- Burping or heartburn
- Headaches
- Sleep disturbances
- Fatigue
- Increased symptoms for women during menstruation

In some cases, people who are lactose intolerant (unable to digest dairy products) may have similar symptoms to IBS. A health care professional can determine whether lactose intolerance is causing your discomfort, or you can perform an at-home test by eliminating dairy from your diet for ten to fourteen days and observing whether the symptoms change or disappear. Those allergic to sorbitol, an artificial sweetener, may also exhibit similar symptoms and can perform a similar at-home test to determine whether sorbitol is the problem.

If a doctor suspects you have IBS, he or she may want to run some tests to rule out the other, more serious diseases mentioned on page 3. You may be asked to provide a stool specimen, get x-rays, undergo an endoscopic examination (where the doctor views the colon through a flexible tube inserted through the anus), or have a barium enema.

Speaking from experience, I can accurately report that these procedures are just a barrel of laughs.

"Orthodox medicine has not found an answer to your complaint. However, luckily for you, I happen to be a quack."

—Richter cartoon caption

Even though the criteria for identifying the condition are straightforward, IBS isn't always at the top of the diagnostic list. A study conducted by the University of California at Los Angeles found that even though 58 percent of the doctors surveyed said IBS is easy to diagnose, 80 percent of those same doctors don't use the Rome criteria for diagnostic purposes. This could explain why most people with the condition go on an average of three doctor visits over the course of three years before they are diagnosed with IBS. Another study, published in October 2000 by Dr. Marvin M. Schuster of Johns Hopkins University, documented that people with IBS have the following in common:

- 40 percent reported intolerable abdominal pain.
- 65 percent plan their day-to-day schedule based on the anticipated use of bathroom facilities.

🍃 53 percent feel that their health limits their activity, whereas only 26 of people without IBS feel the same way.

Ironically, the study also showed that 33 percent of the M.D.'s interviewed believe that IBS is a psychosomatic disorder. In fact, IBS is defined in the Medscape online medical reference dictionary as "a chronic functional disorder of the colon that is of unknown etiology but is commonly considered to be of psychosomatic origin and that is characterized by the secretion and passage of large amounts of mucus, by constipation altering with diarrhea, and by cramping abdominal pain."

Since there is no single known organic cause of the condition, some doctors with the perspective that IBS is psychosomatic give a general message to patients that "it's all in your head." What these doctors are overlooking, however, is that what goes on inside the mind—whether it's positive or negative—almost always contributes to the nature of physical health, distress, or disease (as is explained by mind/body medicine). This relationship is nothing to dismiss, which is why it's important to look at the entire person, not just symptoms. Nevertheless, because of this disparaging attitude, there are doctors who don't consider IBS a condition to take seriously. The vast majority of people who avoid parties, shopping, school, or work would adamantly disagree.

Ruth's Story, Age 32

I stopped eating for a few days when my mother was hospitalized. After she was released, I tried to go back to my normal routine of pizza, fries, and other fast food because before then, I hadn't had any trouble or symptoms at all. My tummy wasn't ready, willing, or able to go back to that diet with me, though. Everything I was used to eating ran right through me. From that point forward, I knew exactly how long it would take me to reach the nearest bathroom no matter where I was, and I never ate within two hours of being in the car. In the past four years, I've only been out to eat four times. Three of those times were painful and embarrassing because I had to leave the table so urgently.

My social life is dead. I use the telephone and Internet to stay in touch with my friends, and even then I have to cut conversations short.

The Physiology of IBS

Even though there are no physical signs of disease or deterioration when the colon is examined, there are physical markers associated with IBS. Studies indicate that the colon muscle of a person with IBS is unusually sensitive, overreacting to both internal and external stimuli such as gas, eating, movement of feces in the intestines, and stress. These influences don't affect bowel function in a person with a normal colon.

The colon is about six feet long and connects the small intestine with the rectum and anus. Each day, about two quarts of liquid matter enter the colon from the small intestine. The major function of the colon is to absorb water, salts, and nutrients from that liquid. After several days of being contained in the colon, most of the nutrients and fluids have been absorbed into the body. The remaining stool then passes through the intestine by a rhythmic pattern to the left side of the colon, where it is stored until a bowel movement occurs. (If you're lucky, that is.)

Nerves, hormones, and electrical activity within the colon control the motility (or contractions) of the muscle and how it propels the stool toward the rectum. During the course of each day, several strong muscle contractions massage the feces ever downward, ultimately resulting in the infamous "BM." A normally functioning colon operates in rhythmic fashion (maybe that's why people who are regular tend to sing and dance about it!), alternating between relaxing and contracting. When a person has IBS, however, the colon has either stronger contractions that last longer or weaker contractions that don't last long enough. In essence, the intestines squeeze the feces too hard and fast, resulting in diarrhea, gas, and bloating, or not hard enough, causing constipation. Both scenarios can lead to abdominal cramping. When chronic diarrhea occurs, it is also difficult for the colon to adequately absorb nutrients, which can eventually lead to a loss of energy and other complications.

The Causes of IBS

According to Western medicine, no one really knows what causes IBS. Experts from the Mayo Foundation for Medical Education say that IBS could be due to changes in the nerves that control sensation or muscle contractions in the bowel, or due to abnormalities in the central nervous system. Since the symptoms tend to worsen when women menstruate, there's also speculation that it is somehow related to hormones.

Bing Lee, Dipl. Ac., who has been practicing acupuncture and Chinese medicine since 1987, has a different stance. He says that there is no *single* cause for this—or any other—imbalance. Rather there may be, and usually are, many factors that contribute to the physiology. As mentioned before, however, isolating the physical malfunctions (or symptoms) doesn't solve the question of what created them. Lee suggests taking a step back and performing an inventory of all areas of your life to assess what may be the source of the distress. We'll guide you through that process later in this book.

Food and IBS

Even though Eastern and Western approaches may differ, both schools of thought agree that symptoms are quite often triggered (not caused) by food-related issues and emotional stress.

FOOD AS AN IRRITANT

It's common among those with IBS to experience symptoms after eating. Overeating, consuming certain foods, and excessive use of laxatives, antibiotics, and other medications can also cause trouble. Some types of food that commonly irritate the colon are:

 Foods high in fat (either animal or vegetable)

 Spicy foods

 Foods that contain caffeine (such as coffee, tea, chocolate, and soda)

Beyond these general categories, specific foods that may cause you distress include:

 Alcohol

 Avocados

 Citrus fruits

 Corn

 Milk and other dairy products

 Sugar

 Wheat

If any of these foods are a pain in the gut to you, stop eating them! See what happens when you eliminate them for a week or so.

Betty's Story, Age 42

When I was diagnosed with IBS about a year ago, my doctor told me to switch to a bland diet. He knows I don't want to control the problem with drugs, so he didn't even mention them to me. Instead, he focused everything on diet. I ate a lot of oatmeal and high-fiber foods, but it didn't make a difference in the cramping. I read some books on diets and nutrition and ended up eliminating all dairy, wheat, animal protein, and sugar, plus most fats. That has left me pretty much with fresh vegetables, a few fruits, some nuts, and soy products. Chocolate is my downfall, and giving that up has been the hardest part. But whenever I sneak some, I have these terrible cramps. It gets depressing, though, when you go out and you can't eat anything you love. Things are a little better, but I'm not sure if this is really what needs to change.

FOOD AS MEDICINE

If you've consulted a physician about your symptoms, chances are you've been advised to change your diet in the hopes that doing so will relieve discomfort and normalize your stool. This helps some people (but not everyone—remember, there is no magic bullet) and is a convenient, inexpensive, and manageable option for everyone. We recommend that if you haven't already tried these food-related suggestions, you give them a shot. Who knows—food may be part of the problem.

> "Sour, sweet, bitter, pungent, all must be tasted."
>
> —Chinese proverb

Keep a food journal. The easiest way to determine whether a food triggers your symptoms is to record your habits. Write down everything you eat and at what time. Take note when a specific food causes trouble. Jot down how long after eating the problem occurred, exactly what you experienced (such as abdominal pain resulting in diarrhea or bad gas and bloating), how long the symptoms lasted, and how severe they were. Becoming aware of eating habits and specific food triggers can enlighten you about new ways to eat (such as more slowly, perhaps), how much to eat, and most important, what to avoid eating. Keep in mind that it's normal to have colon contractions about 30 to 60 minutes after you eat.

Reduce your saturated fat intake. Due to the high calorie content, fat causes more contractions in the colon than less-fatty or lower-calorie foods. Healthy fats are necessary and good (more on this in Chapter Nine; see page 146), but you should stay clear of the saturated fats found in butter, peanut butter, fatty cuts of animal protein, and whole-milk dairy products. Instead, choose monounsaturated fats found in olive oil, canola oil, peanut oil, peanuts, cashews, and almonds.

Supplement with essential fatty acids (EFAs). Shoot for omega-3 and omega-6 essential fatty acids. Both create prostaglandins—hormonelike substances that help manage healthy cardiovascular, immune, nervous, and reproductive systems. Although omega-3 sports more linolenic acid than omega-6 fats, both contain important properties for improved health due to their inflammation-reducing abilities. There are myriad other health reasons to keep both omegas running through your colon. But in the case of some-one suffering from IBS, eating plenty of cod, herring, mackerel, tuna, sardines, and salmon, or supplementing with borage, evening primrose, or flaxseed oil, may make your gut—and your spirits—happier. That's because EFAs have also been found to improve depression, the dour stepsister of IBS.

Fill up on fiber. There are two kinds of fiber: soluble (meaning it dissolves in water) and insoluble. The soluble kind helps relieve both diarrhea and constipation, but insoluble fiber can worsen diarrhea. Those who suffer from loose stools should avoid getting fiber from fruits, vegetables, whole-grain breads, cereals, pasta, and rice. Instead, turn to the soluble form found in oat bran or psyllium (natural vegetable fiber), which is available in over-the-counter supplements. Taking psyllium on a regular basis may also lower cholesterol and help with weight loss. But don't take it within two hours of other supplements or medications, as it can postpone absorption of some substances into the bloodstream. Also, if you develop a rash, itch, or have trouble breathing, stop taking psyllium immediately! That's an allergic reaction that warrants medical attention. To begin, we recommend that you take one teaspoon of psyllium once or twice a day mixed with water. After your body has become accustomed to the additional fiber, follow the package directions for usage. Regardless of what type of fiber you ingest, take it with as much water as you can, preferably six to eight glasses per day, and introduce it gradually, as it can be a little rough on your body.

The reason fiber helps certain people is because it absorbs water from the intestines and keeps moisture in the stool, thus preventing those pesky, hard turds that are reluctant to leave the warmth of your body. Fiber also fills out your colon with a bulking effect that helps prevent painful spasms. The downside of bulking up, however, is that it may cause bloating or gas—and in some people, it may even worsen their overall symptoms. Don't let this scare you. Nothing works for everyone, and the only way to know if fiber can help is to give it a try. Keep in mind that it's normal to have some gas and bloating (hey, what's new?) during the first few weeks of increased fiber consumption. Stick with it for a week or two. If things don't settle down, ease up on the fiber and try another tactic.

Avoid gas-producing foods. If you're one of those gaseous people (I won the award for most prolific pooter in high school), then stop eating foods that cause gas. Avoid beans, broccoli, cauliflower, cucumbers, lentils, onions, peas, and leafy green veggies. Be mindful that your system is unique and may be sensitive to foods that other people can eat without a hitch. Garlic, for instance, turns me into a stinky noise machine, but my family can eat it by the bushel and sleep through the night without a sound.

Eat smaller meals, spread throughout the day. Smaller meals are easier on your already-hard-at-work digestive system. Eating four to six meals throughout the day may let your stomach take it easy, and therefore reduce symptoms.

Even if you've tried these measures in the past and have had no luck in alleviating your symptoms, it's always wise to avoid processed and refined foods. Try to stick with the foods that are as true to nature as possible.

The Effects of Emotional Stress

Valerie's Story, Age 29

I feel my symptoms are connected with emotional problems. Before I was diagnosed with IBS, I always thought it was something I was doing to myself. I grew up with a verbally abusive father. He constantly yelled at me at the dinner table, and I could never continue to eat once he started in on me. He drilled it into me that I would never amount to anything because I was female, so I worked extra hard on my grades and in sports to try and please him. But with every perfect grade and trophy, he made it clear that I still wasn't good enough. He taught me that I was boring, unattractive, untalented, and stupid. In my teen years, I started to starve myself to avoid having the pains in my abdomen.

Eventually, I just didn't want to eat anymore. But I couldn't live that way, so I got some counseling. I did some modeling. I graduated with awards and a 3.9 G.P.A. Now, I'm a very happy and successful person. My emotional problems are behind me, although I still live with the symptoms.

Stress is part of life. It's usually rooted in fretting about the past, worrying about the future, or going about life without meeting important personal needs. It kicks up after a bad night's sleep or because of financial woes, a dictatorial boss, screaming kids, too much partying, incontinent dogs, hunger, frustration, loneliness, lethargy, a bad date, a sense of being overwhelmed, boredom—the list could fill this book. But there's one simple truth about stress: It's more predictable than either death or taxes.

You may already be aware of an intimate relationship between your colon and stress. When I was a teenager, the slightest scary thing could set off a reaction: being called to the principal's office, an angry tone in my father's voice, a bad grade, or even a flirtatious glance from a cute guy. That's right—good stuff can be stressful, too! Oh, the times when I had to make a beeline to the john with only seconds to spare because of some new source of stress. This is a familiar scenario for people with IBS, and it can turn into a nightmare when there's a long line at a public restroom. In those cases, it's best to turn on the charm, fall on bended knee, and beg for mercy from the people in front of you. I've done it on more occasions than I want to remember.

"Are you stressed? Are you so busy getting to the future that the present is reduced to a means of getting there? Stress is caused by being 'here' but wanting to be 'there,' or being in the present but wanting to be in the future. It's a split that tears you apart inside. To create and live with such an inner split is insane. The fact that everyone else is doing it doesn't make it any less insane."

—Eckhart Tolle
The Power of Now

Since most of us don't know how to eliminate stress from life, the only other choice is to learn how to deal with it. In Chapters Two and Eight (pages 32 and 137), we'll discusses some strategies for accomplishing this.

> "All men have an instinct for conflict: at least, all healthy men."
>
> —Hilaire Belloc
> *The Silence of the Sea*

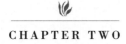

CHAPTER TWO

Treating IBS in the Western World

Linda's Story, Age 36

When I first went to the doctor about the abdominal pains I was having, they thought it was a gynecological problem. They conducted five laparoscopies on me and determined that I had a mild case of endometriosis. The pain didn't stop, so I went to a gastroenterologist who did a lower and upper GI sigmoidoscopy and colonoscopy, an IVP kidney ultrasound, a gallbladder test, and finally a complete hysterectomy. It didn't work. The pain is still there and the symptoms are getting worse.

Years ago, doctors might conduct surgeries such as laparoscopies, hysterectomies, and appendectomies on patients who were desperate for relief from the symptoms of irritable bowel syndrome. These days, most doctors wouldn't even think of surgery as an option—although tragically, some continue to.

Rather than surgery, in today's world pharmaceutical drugs are the tools of choice with which M.D.'s typically treat IBS. Remaining true to the culture of the world's best medical schools, most M.D.'s rely on a variety of pills, capsules, tinctures, syrups, or other forms of synthetic drugs to find relief for their patients. Plus, by doing that, they keep the pharmaceutical industry *very* healthy—a die-hard tradition for American medical doctors ever since the politics of medicine created these strange bedfellows. That's because the long-standing, accepted approach to teaching and practicing medicine has been with drugs. It's no secret that the Food and Drug Administration (FDA) is closely aligned with the pharmaceutical industry. For example, it's not uncommon for someone from the pharmaceutical industry to occupy a position with the FDA or for someone to get promises of a prestigious job with a pharmaceutical company after leaving the FDA. The FDA is an agency that approves or disapproves of the medicines doctors give their patients, so the obvious choice for the FDA is to favor medicines that make money for the pharmaceutical industry.

Historically, if an M.D. wanted to explore alternative means of healing, he or she risked being ostracized by peers or no longer per-mitted to practice in local hospitals. This type of reaction prevented many M.D.'s from even considering using alternative medicine, and it certainly made it harder for patients wanting alternative treatment to find it. Fortunately, with consumer demand, the closed-minded atti-tude about alternative approaches in traditional medical circles is slowly opening.

Even so, the tradition in medicine is to turn to drugs, but rarely do doctors pull cures from the medicine cabinet. And too often, the drugs themselves create a list of new ailments in IBS patients.

Take me, for example. After privately dealing with several pain-ful—and at times terrifying—bouts of IBS, I finally confessed to my mother that I was living a double life. In one part of my life, I was a functioning student, daughter, and friend who experienced the manic joys and melodramas normally associated with being a teenager. The other part of my life was lived out in the bathroom, where I was a prisoner of war, under brutal attack by invisible forces that captured my intestines, tortured them, and gave only sporadic relief in the form of firm feces.

With horror in her heart at what might be wrong, Mom took me to a doctor who ran me through the usual battery of tests over the course of several weeks and concluded that I had IBS. His solution was to prescribe belladonna, a tincture made from opium.

In those days, the idea of trying a little opium sounded exotic and, frankly, appealing. I had visions of floating through my days at school, stress free, pain free, and with a glow that would cast a new, more enjoyable light on the tedium of my studies. So as the wise doctor instructed, I ingested several droppers-full of the drug each day, comfortable with his promises that the pain in my gut would subside and my own fantasy that all was well.

I don't remember if the pain from the IBS subsided. I do remember that my bowels continued to inspire lines from opposing songs such as "I'm stuck in the middle with you" and "You're runnin' too fast, you're runnin' too fast!" I don't remember a less-distended stomach. I do remember maintaining my reputation as a proficient pooter. Mostly, however, I was so drowsy, thick-headed, enervated, and forgetful that I could hardly stay awake at school, much less function effectively. Mom obviously liked living with a tamer teen, and she urged me to continue with the medication. But it was clear to me that by anesthetizing myself with opium, I was going to miss out on the joy and vitality I had experienced in my life before taking it. Much to my mother's chagrin, I stopped taking the prescription one week after starting it, and I began opening my mind to new ways of easing the pain and calming my upset tummy.

"Words are, of course, the most powerful drug used by mankind."

—Rudyard Kipling

Some may argue that being sleepy is better than being in pain. My doctor certainly thought it was an appropriate choice. It's true that the side effects I experienced weren't life threatening or, to some people's thinking, even serious. Still, while under the influence of the drug, I felt as though I was captive in a glass bubble filled with a heavy fog. I could see through the haze just enough to perform, but being in the bubble kept me at arms' length from truly engaging in my life. In short, I felt cut off from the thrill of life, the richness, the wonder. That was a side effect I wasn't willing to live with.

Some people with IBS have found relief through taking drugs without experiencing uncomfortable side effects, and for them we are happy. Even so, it's important to be aware of the potential side effects of any drug you take—especially since the drug could create more serious (even life-threatening) conditions than the imbalance it is treating.

The Drug Tradeoff and the Dance of Finding Relief

Angie's Story, Age 39

I've gone from one drug to another. They put me on Tagamet. It didn't work. They put me on Prevacid. It didn't work. I tried Prilosec, but it made the constipation worse. I went on Zantac, and I experienced chest pains. They said I was depressed, so they put me on Paxil. I could no longer climax during sex, and then heart palpitations started. My body is so tired. I'm so tired. I'm wondering what to fight for anymore.

In 1997, taking prescription drugs to fight aches, pains, and illnesses roped in a staggering $60 billion in this country. Prescription drugs are approved by the Food and Drug Administration (FDA) before being distributed, but 51 percent of them create adverse side effects that aren't detected until people start taking them. Sadly, that results in more than 140,000 deaths every year. According to Thomas J. Moore, author of *Prescription for Disaster: The Hidden Dangers in Your Medicine Cabinet*, that's four times the number of people murdered each year and twice the number of people that die in car accidents. He further states that 1 million people are severely injured by prescription drugs each year and 2 million more are harmed yearly by drugs taken while in the hospital.

> "A faithful friend is the medicine of life."
>
> —Ecclesiasticus

We're not saying you should never take pharmaceutical drugs. They can provide desperately needed relief in many critical situations. They've done wonders for emergency medicine and dealing with terminal diseases such as cancer. But we do think that finding alternatives to drugs for chronic, less-threatening conditions such as IBS is wise. Let's look at why, starting with my favorite example: belladonna.

Belladonna and its derivatives, such as atropine, clidinium, dicylomine, glycopyrrolate, homatropine, hyoscyamine, and mepenzolate, are considered antispasmodics. Among other things, these drugs are supposed to relieve cramps or spasms of the stomach, intestines, and bladder, and in conjunction with antacids, decrease the distress related to peptic ulcers. The United States Pharmacopeial Convention claims that some of these drugs also help prevent nausea, vomiting, and motion sickness. At first glance, it seems reasonable that doctors might prescribe antispasmodic medications for those afflicted with IBS.

Upon reading the fine print about the risks associated with them, however, the reasons that these drugs are prescribed become blurry. Common side effects include constipation (hey, wait, that was my *symptom!*), decrease in sweating, and a dry mouth, nose, throat, or skin. Less common side effects include bloating (another one of my symptoms) blurred vision, difficulty urinating, difficulty swallowing, drowsiness (no kidding), headaches, sensitivity to light, loss of memory (yep), nausea, vomiting (isn't that what it's supposed to prevent?), unusual tiredness, and weakness (this one is true). Rare side effects include confusion, dizziness, light-headedness, fainting, eye pain, skin rashes, and hives.

Ironically, belladonna makes you sweat less while it increases your heart rate. This can cause your body temperature to rise, which can be dangerous if you exercise and become overheated. I was a teenager back when I was taking it, busily playing sports every day and soothing my tired body in a hot bath every night. Although precautions state that overheating from exercise or hot baths or saunas may result in heat stroke or severe dizziness, my doctor never mentioned that I should be careful of that. Nor did he mention that belladonna could be habit forming and that I should gradually stop using the drug to avoid typical withdrawal symptoms such as vomiting, sweating, and dizziness. Since my reaction to belladonna already included severe drowsiness and dizziness, it probably didn't matter that I stopped cold turkey after my miserable week of living in the glass bubble.

David's Story, Age 28

The only thing I've found that relieves my diarrhea is methadone. It may sound crazy, but I go to a methadone clinic for my fix, and it works. I know it's addictive, but I'd rather be addicted to drugs than live my life running to the bathroom every ten minutes. Maybe someday I'll find some other way, but my doctor agrees that this is okay for now.

Looking closer at the other drugs commonly prescribed for IBS, it's no wonder that so many people end up feeling more frustrated than relieved after using them. Again—there are people for whom these drugs work. Terrific. But if they haven't worked for you, don't throw up your hands and feel like you're alone. Given the many side effects, it's no wonder that you may not have had good luck! Here's a quick rundown of some of the more commonly prescribed drugs and what they were actually developed to treat, plus some concerns you may or may not find listed on the packaging.

"Who shall decide when doctors disagree?"

—Alexander Pope

Tagamet (cimetidine), Pepcid (famotidine), and Zantac (ranitidine hydrochloride). Doctors very often recommend these

over-the-counter drugs to IBS patients—even though they were created for and are more commonly used to treat acid indigestion and
symptoms related to ulcers. Known as H2 receptor antagonists, their
job is to prevent histamines from releasing certain chemicals into
your stomach (such as hydrochloric acid, which aids in digestion). By
blocking this ability, stomach acids are reduced, which can momen-
tarily prevent acid indigestion in those IBS sufferers who experience
it. Problem is, stomach acids don't cause IBS, so popping these pills
won't do the ultimate job of relieving your symptoms.

**Reglan (metoclopramide hydrochloride) and Propulsid
(cisapride).** These drugs are gastrointestinal stimulants, which
means they create intestinal contractions to move food through the
GI tract. They are most commonly prescribed for patients with
severe heartburn. Reglan is also used to prevent nausea in people
undergoing chemotherapy.

Taking Propulsid with other medications has been known to
cause heart arrhythmias. Consequently, the FDA has warned that
anyone with heart disease and a host of other diseases should not
take it. According to Natural Medicine Online, this warning was
issued after approximately 70 Propulsid users died and 200 others
reported heart problems (some life-threatening) since Propulsid's
release in 1993. And think about it: If it's a stimulant, what happens
if your symptoms include diarrhea?

Prilosec (omeprazole). Another drug targeted at decreasing
excessive amounts of stomach acid, Prilosec is prescribed primarily
for those with ulcers. (Again, this is not a symptom that people with
IBS struggle with.) Although still under investigation, studies indicate that it may be carcinogenic.

Lomotil (diphenoxylate hydrochloride). This drug slows
movement within the intestines, which helps prevent diarrhea. It's
mostly prescribed for treatment of diarrhea. Ironically, one of the
side effects of this drug is constipation. And although overdosing on
any drug can be dangerous, if you make that mistake with Lomotil,
it will kill you.

Most M.D.'s are doing the best they can and earnestly want to
help their patients. But when you learn about some of the side

effects (such as diarrhea, abdominal pain, constipation, bloating, gas, indigestion, and intestinal blockage) that can occur by taking drugs commonly prescribed for IBS, you may rightly question why these drugs are ever prescribed for the condition.

There are many drugs prescribed to treat IBS-related symptoms, including those we've already mentioned. But none work effectively and safely for the majority of people who take them for IBS. Meanwhile, there are cases where the FDA has clearly made mistakes by approving drugs for IBS, only to discover their toxic and sometimes fatal impact on users. One such drug was alosetron hydrochloride.

In early 2000, doctors thought alosetron hydrochloride (known as Lotronex) was the answer for women who suffer from IBS. Men couldn't take it (they absorb alosetron faster than women do, and scientists never determined an effective dose), but 300,000 women turned to it for relief. Although researchers weren't entirely sure why, the drug was indeed successful in slowing intestinal movement. Users found relief after 12 weeks of taking Lotronex, but once they stopped taking it, all symptoms returned.

Unfortunately, the side effects of this drug proved highly dangerous. Common side effects included severe constipation, which required some users to turn to laxatives and large amounts of fiber for relief. Other patients acquired acute colitis (inflammation of the large intestines, a far more serious condition than IBS), bloody diarrhea, or worsening of abdominal pain. Only eight months after it was released, the FDA received notice that three deaths were associated with the drug due to severe complications that occurred from subsequent development of colitis. There were also forty-nine cases of ischemic colitis (inflammation of the large bowel from lack of blood flow) and twenty-one cases of severe constipation among users. It was immediately pulled from the shelves and is no longer available.

"We don't know a millionth of one percent about anything."

—Thomas Edison

Antidepressants, anxiety drugs, and barbiturates are also frequently prescribed for symptoms of IBS. Some argue that these drugs help what ails the gut even though they target the psychological life of the patient. The deduction: If you're more relaxed about life, you will probably have fewer attacks in the colon. Also, many people with IBS *do* experience depression—so why not get a little help from the brain-chemical medicine cabinet? On the surface, this seems like a sensible approach to helping with the problem. Taking a closer look at the common side effects of this type of drug, however, may change your mind.

Elavil (amitriptyline hydrochloride). This antidepressant increases the chemicals that provide nerve transmissions within the brain. The result: no more depression. It's also used to treat bulimia, migraines, chronic pain, and certain symptoms associated with multiple sclerosis. The list of *common* side effects is as lengthy as several squares of toilet paper and includes, among other things, constipation, sexual impairment, diarrhea, and stomach upset. This drug is habit forming and should be gradually withdrawn from the system.

Librax (chlordiazepoxide hydrochloride with clidinium bromide). This is an anti-anxiety drug and anticholinergic, which means (like others above) it reduces the production of stomach acids and slows down activity in the gastrointestinal tract. Meanwhile, it depresses the central nervous system, which reduces anxiety. Some side effects include decreased sex drive, constipation, abdominal pain, bloating, and gas.

Donnatal (phenobarbitol). This is a barbiturate, anticholinergic, and antispasmodic. Like its cousins, it slows down bowel movements and reduces the production of stomach acids. It's often given to treat abdominal pains and cramping. Again, you could wallpaper your bathroom with the list of common side effects. A few of them include a bloated feeling and constipation. Less common side effects could leave you gassy or depressed. And, say the writers of *The Complete Guide to Pills*, this drug is habit forming and should not be taken if you have "diseases that block the gastrointestinal tract."

Prozac (fluoxetine hydrochloride). Probably the most widely recognized name in antidepressants. Eli Lilly, which produces the drug, boasts that 34.5 million people in more than 100 countries, including 17 million Americans, take it. But according to the FDA, Prozac is associated with more hospitalization deaths and serious adverse side effects than any other drug in America! That's depressing, if you ask me. Prozac is a selective serotonin reuptake inhibitor (SSRI) that inhibits the activity of neurons that control the intestines. It also increases the concentration of chemicals that transmit information from nerve to nerve within the brain, which helps with depression, difficulty concentrating, and other psychological challenges. Common side effects include diarrhea. Rare side effects go from here to the county line and include constipation, inflammation of the stomach lining, bloody diarrhea, colitis, duodenal ulcers, enlarged abdomen, inability to control bowel movements, gas, inflammation of the small intestine, stomach ulcers, and death.

Paxil (paroxetine hydrochloride). Like Prozac, this SSRI increases the concentration of chemicals that control nerve transmission in the brain. It's used to treat serious, ongoing depression. Common side effects include but are not limited to abdominal pain, constipation, diarrhea, fluid retention, gas, stomach pain, decreased sex drive, and vertigo. Less common side effects take up pages; among them are belching, bloody diarrhea, indigestion, inflammation of the stomach, rectal bleeding, vomiting, dark and tarry stools, impacted stool, inability to control bowel movements, and peptic or stomach ulcers.

Ben's Story, Age 28

I've had chronic diarrhea for about ten years. I always felt cheated because of it. I was too young when I got it, and I'm too young to still have it. Last year, my doctor told me he thought I should go on an antidepressant. I said, "Don't you think it's normal for a young guy like me to get depressed over having to spend his life in the crapper?" He said drugs would help, so I went on Elavil. Well, the doctor was wrong. Things got worse. I gained weight, I was always thirsty, and I was walking around like a zombie because I was so tired. One day, my girlfriend couldn't wake me up—even tugging on my shoulders. She finally sprayed me with some water and I woke up. But my sex drive didn't. I lost it. I thought having to live in the crapper was bad—nothing compares to being unable to have sex.

The Last Resort: Alternative Therapies

"It is common sense to take a method and try it. If it fails, admit it frankly and try another. But above all, try something."

—Franklin D. Roosevelt

Weary from the side effects, lack of positive results, or expense of these drugs, many people have turned to alternative medicine in an attempt to manage their IBS. Most of these therapies are available without a prescription through local health care professionals or good health food stores; cost far less than pharmaceutical drugs; and have few, if any, side effects. Even so, we'll remind you again that there is no single solution for everyone, so if you've tried one therapy without success, it doesn't mean you should lock yourself in the loo and throw away the key. That's why we're covering everything, starting with simple methods and leading up to traditional Chinese medicine (TCM), which we think offers the most promise.

There are basically two common approaches to working with IBS from an alternative point of view: one is with herbal or homeopathic supplements and the other is through stress-reduction strategies.

SUPPLEMENTS

For years, Americans accustomed to prescription drugs have erroneously believed that herbs are an archaic treatment and therefore useless. Either that, or they figured using herbs for medicinal purposes was something new and unproven. Neither is true. Soon you'll discover how prevalent herbs have been in TCM and other ancient healing arts throughout history and the world. What is new, however, is that herbal medicines are finally being paid the respect they deserve among America's allopathic doctors.

I single out Americans because in other places around the world, the medicinal properties of herbs have been studied and documented for years. In most European countries, herbal treatment is commonplace. In Germany, for example, it's typical that a doctor would automatically suggest and provide chamomile for digestive disorders such as IBS. Likewise, only 2 percent of the German population takes Prozac for depression, while 50 percent battle the blues with St.-John's-wort (which works, in most cases, without side effects).

Furthermore, European companies and even governments fund the study of herbal treatments. Back in 1978, the German government established Commission E, a committee of experts that evaluates the safety and efficacy of medicinal herbs. The experts include physicians, pharmacists, nonmedical practitioners, toxologists, pharmacologists, and biostatisticians. By 1995, Commission E had evaluated 360 herbs and 391 parts of herbs that it believed could be beneficial to humans.

Although herbal research is more prevalent in America than it used to be, America's medical community typically ignores these studies. The reason? Natural products, such as foods, herbs, spices, vitamins, and so forth, cannot be patented. Hence, few companies will spend the money necessary for research and development of an herbal remedy. It simply wouldn't pay off. This is true even though about 10 percent of what people spend at the health food store goes toward purchasing medicinal or raw herbs.

Instead, our pharmaceutical companies spend their money on the research and development of synthetic drugs, which they can patent and turn into significant profits. To illustrate, the Health Care Financing Administration says that sales of prescription drugs nearly doubled from 1993 to 1998. In this country, the tradition of medicine is tightly wound up in making money—lots of it—sometimes at the expense of an ailing population. When you consider the amount of money people spend on these drugs, couple that with side effects, and acknowledge that the drugs are treating symptoms rather than causes, you find that it's quite a price to pay. Especially when so many alternative treatments can be equally or more effective than drugs, cost far less, and spare the patient from debilitating side effects. Even so, studying and developing synthetic drugs clearly take precedence over natural and herbal supplements.

Though you're not likely to learn about them from your primary care physician, many herbs and supplements can be used to treat IBS. We'll elaborate on the use of some of these treatments later in the book, but here's a quick overview.

If you opt to try one or a combination of these remedies, be sure to consult with either your medical doctor or a qualified health care practitioner before you begin. Herbal medicines can be very powerful, and there have been incidents—although far fewer than with drugs—of side effects. Be especially mindful that if you are on prescription drugs, some herbs can interfere with their effectiveness, or there may be contraindications to using the treatments simultaneously.

Note: Pregnant women should always consult a physician before taking any supplements. Some are uterine stimulants that could cause miscarriage.

Arrowroot. Recent studies indicate that arrowroot is an effective treatment for diarrhea and has a long-term positive effect on constipation while easing abdominal pain.

Artichoke extract. It's little known that this delightful little morsel of a plant helps the formation and flow of bile. When there's more free-flowing bile running through your system, your body works more effectively by softening stools and cleaning out microorganisms from the small intestines. This adds up to a healthier gut, and for some, it relieves symptoms of IBS.

Chamomile. Taken as a tea or a tincture, this anti-inflammatory and antispasmodic reduces gas and is a good all-around gut calmer. It also helps with insomnia and general tension. Avoid it if you're pregnant, though, as it stimulates the uterus.

Enzymes. Bacteria feeds on fermented sugar and produces two basic by-products: methane gas and acidic acid. These both result in symptoms of IBS: flatulence and inflamed bowels, or mucus or blood in the bowels, respectively. Enzymes can help digest sugar, which cuts down on the unwanted byproducts.

Fennel. Ingested as a tea or by chewing the seeds (you've probably seen them in big glass bowls at many Indian restaurants), this herb helps relieve gas and indigestion. It, too, is a uterine stimulant, so if you're pregnant, stay clear!

Homeopathics. Even though homeopathic treatments can be purchased at health food stores, we recommend that you work with a health care practitioner before investing in these concoctions. Based on a science that recognizes how *like treats like*, homeopathics actually introduce a small dose of whatever problem is currently occurring in the body, which causes the body's natural healing mechanisms to kick in. Some people have had good results relieving tension and easing the symptoms of IBS by using homeopathics.

Marshmallow. Taken as a tincture, this sweet herb is good for reducing inflammation of the mucous membranes of the digestive tract. Pregnant women are safe with this one.

Myrrh. Used for many medicinal purposes, this herb acts as an antibacterial agent in the stomach and stimulates the flow of gastric juices. And—you guessed it—it stimulates the uterus.

Peppermint oil. Some people have gotten good results from this natural antispasmodic that relaxes and smoothes the intestinal muscles. It reportedly reduces gas, bloating, and abdominal pain. Enteric-coated peppermint oil is best because the menthol isn't released in the stomach; rather, it and other active ingredients are released in the colon, which is where soothing is most needed. Beware that peppermint can make symptoms worse in some people, and it has been known to aggravate heartburn.

Valerian: Widely used to help relieve insomnia (although you shouldn't mix it with other sleeping aids), this herb is also good for relieving gas, relaxing muscles, calming anxiety, and soothing pain. Don't use it for more than three weeks continuously, or you may experience headaches or heart palpitations. It's not recommended for pregnant women, and it can also interfere with certain medications, so talk to a doctor before taking it.

Yarrow. When you drink this in tea form, it stimulates the flow of bile, calms muscles, and relieves spasms. It can also be used as a diuretic. Rare allergic reactions show up as skin rash. It is also a uterine stimulant.

"Better is a dinner of herbs where love is, than a salted ox and hatred therewith."

—Proverbs 15:17

🌿

Alternative Medicine Veers into the Mainstream

According to the *Journal of the American Medical Association*, 33.8 percent of the population used alternative therapies in 1990; that percentage increased to 42.1 percent in 1997. Therapies of choice included herbal medicine, acupuncture, exercise, massage, megavitamins, self-help groups, folk remedies, energy healing, relaxation techniques, chiropractic, imagery, spiritual healing, commercial weight-loss programs, lifestyle diets (such as macrobiotics), biofeedback, hypnosis, homeopathy, and prayer. Alternative therapies were used most frequently for chronic conditions such as backaches, anxiety, depression, and headaches.

In 1997, approximately 15 million adults took prescription drugs while supplementing with either herbal remedies or vitamins, but only 38.5 percent of those who used alternative therapy told their medical doctor about it.

There were an estimated 629 million visits to alternative care practitioners in 1997—exceeding the total number of visits to primary care physicians, and a considerable increase from the 427 million visits in 1990. Slightly more than 58 percent of patients paid for the alternative care out-of-pocket. The cost for those alternative services was approximately $21.2 billion, with about $12 billion paid out-of-pocket. This exceeds the 1997 out-of-pocket expenditures for all U.S. hospitalizations. A conservative estimate of the total expenditure for all types of alternative treatments (including those not requiring a health care practitioner) adds up to $27 billion, comparable to the out-of-pocket expenditures for all U.S. physician services.

STRESS-REDUCTION STRATEGIES

Many people believe, and now studies agree, that when you combine stress management techniques with physical treatment, you stand a better chance of feeling good and reducing IBS symptoms. A study conducted through the department of medicine at Humboldt University in Berlin and published in the May 2000 *American Journal of Gastroenterology* reported that there is "evidence that the combination of medical treatment plus . . . behavioral treatment is superior to medical treatment alone in therapy of IBS."

In the study, one segment of people with IBS attended ten sessions of therapy lasting for one hour each over a ten-week period. In the sessions, they were provided with information about IBS, as well as an analysis of their own unique symptoms; training in muscle relaxation, coping strategies, and problem solving; and assertiveness training. After the study was concluded, those patients who underwent therapy felt more in control of their health and agreed that they had a better quality of life than those patients who did not partake in behavioral therapy.

> "Give a man a fish and he will eat for a day. Teach a man to fish and he will eat for the rest of his life."
>
> —Chinese proverb

Working with a counselor to figure out how to cope with stress is one approach to living a more relaxed life. Other suggestions include:

Mediation. There are thousands of books, tapes, and classes that can teach you a variety of methods for meditation. Even without formal meditation techniques, it can help tremendously to take 20 minutes out of your day, sit or lie down, and simply quit "doing." Here's a challenge: During those 20 minutes, try not to think of anything from the past or the future. That can get your mind off your troubles!

Biofeedback. This technique for relaxation teaches people to control involuntary functions of the body. For example, when you feel your gut stirring up trouble, exercising what you learn from biofeedback enables you to calm your gut, which eases the pain and gives you enough time to get to a bathroom. It's usually taught in hospitals and medical centers and through private counselors.

Exercise. Everyone knows exercise is an essential element for staying healthy—both physically and psychologically. But are you *doing* it regularly? Here are some good reasons you should: Exercising firms your abdominal muscles, while also triggering intestinal contractions that keep things moving smoothly in the GI tract. You don't have to run marathons, either. Walking is fine, but anything that works up a mild sweat will stimulate digestion. Need another reason? Those who exercise regularly say the severity of their symptoms is reduced dramatically. Shoot for 20 minutes of exercise three times a week, minimum!

Deep breathing. Some people find that when they learn to breathe from the diaphragm instead of shallowly, from the chest, it helps promote relaxation. Consequently, it also helps relax abdominal muscles.

Yoga. This ancient form of deep breathing and stretching strengthens muscles, improves circulation, releases endorphins, and has an overall wonderfully calming effect.

Reiki. This Japanese art of healing is based on a philosophy that the laying of hands on different parts of the body can balance body, mind, and spirit by unblocking energy and helping the body reach homeostasis by healing itself. It's gentle and relaxing, and for some, it works wonders.

Massage therapy. There are many types of massage, but all are reputed to improve circulation to muscles, decrease stress, and calm muscle pain and spasms. A good massage also sets free those nifty endorphins, which make you feel good and give you a better night's sleep.

Hypnotherapy. In 1995, the National Institutes of Health determined that hypnotherapy is an effective treatment for IBS. And you don't even need someone else there with you! A study published in *Integrative Medicine Communications* suggested that twelve weeks of self-hypnotherapy using audiotapes about relaxation techniques helped reduce abdominal pain and bloating. That's the good news. The bad news is that hypnotherapy seems to work more for people under 50 years of age. Only about one-fourth of those over 50 who suffer from IBS find hypnotherapy helpful.

Now that you've got the rundown on some alternative approaches, let's take an in-depth look at the one we believe you'll find most useful. Chapter Three will more thoroughly explore traditional Chinese medicine and how it can help you reclaim your life from IBS.

"When in doubt, make a fool of yourself. There is a microscopically thin line between being brilliantly creative and acting like the most gigantic idiot on earth. So what the hell, leap."

—Cynthia Heimel

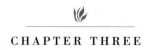

CHAPTER THREE

Understanding Traditional Chinese Medicine

Grasping the basics of traditional Chinese medicine (TCM) may take a few minutes. It's good to know just a smidge about it, though, so you can move into treatment with an understanding of your role in healing. This knowledge will also provide you with an understanding of why a TCM practitioner asks and does what she does. It can show you how pieces from your life may fit into the puzzle of why you're experiencing IBS in the first place. To sum it up, there's more to this than sitting on a cold, metal table wearing an embarrassing smock and talking about constipation, diarrhea, and gas.

> "He who asks a question is a fool for five minutes; he who does not ask a question remains a fool forever."
>
> —Chinese proverb

The Ancient Art of TCM

When medicines were first being developed in Asia nearly 4,000 years ago, the definition of health and wellness encompassed a complex dynamic. Finding cures to illnesses, therefore, was also a multifaceted process. With influences from the places that are now China, Japan, Korea, Tibet, and Vietnam, the concepts themselves included elements of Taoism, Buddhism, and Confucianism, but they were mostly drawn from Taoist philosophy. Those ingredients combined to make a holistic definition of health that looked not only to the physical body but also to spiritual, social, political, and philosophical influences. These are a few aspects that American medicine tends to overlook, and they represent the biggest difference between how the West and East approach healing.

The concepts were first documented in the *Treatise on Diseases Caused by Cold Factors* during the Han dynasty in China between 206 B.C. and 220 A.D. That was followed by what are now considered two of the classics chronicling TCM, *Nei Jing* and *Nan Jing*, written between 100 B.C and 200 A.D. Other valuable texts were written, including the *Yellow Emperor's Inner Classic* (penned about 200 B.C.), but it wasn't until the Ming dynasty in China (1368–1644 A.D) that the *Meteria Medica* or *Pen Tspao Kang Mu* was compiled. It illuminated nearly 2,000 different kinds of medicines, as well as the core concepts behind the TCM way of healing. The Ming dynasty hosted the golden years of Chinese medicine, after which it fell into the background as folklore. Even so, it gradually spread across the continents, coming to America in the nineteenth century. Today, the original concepts conceived thousands of years ago remain the blueprint for TCM, although the practice has evolved into many different branches.

At first glance, you could think that an approach to medicine developed so many millennia ago sounds a bit, well . . . outdated. It's ancient, all right. But that's why it's rife not only with positive results but also with wisdom. It's been tried, tested, reworked, and perfected for so long that current technologies are as yet unable to discern why much of it works at all. What's more, Sheng Nung, the legendary Chinese father of agriculture and TCM itself, could argue that spending his lifetime testing hundreds of different plants for their nutritional and medicinal qualities has yielded lasting and undeniable health benefits to millions of people for generations.

Since pharmaceutical companies are not going to research them, we should be thankful that Mr. Nung did and simply acknowledge that time has done nothing less than refine his research to a masterful and healing art form.

For a long time it was a relatively neglected art, however, as it was considered folk medicine even in China, and other, more modern approaches to health took the limelight. But in 1949, the People's Republic of China decided to merge TCM with the newer methodologies, thus making health care available to all members of society. In America, meanwhile, TCM had found a place to prosper in the Chinese districts of bigger cities, but it was mostly unknown outside of those neighborhoods. It didn't "come out" until 1971, when James Reston, a *New York Times* reporter, wrote about his own experience with it. While covering a Ping-Pong match in Beijing, he was afflicted with appendicitis. After his operation in a local hospital, they used acupuncture to treat his post-surgical pain. Reston came back home feeling healthy and happy, with a front-page story titled "I Have Seen the Past, and It Works!"

Serendipitously, that was when many Americans were looking for alternatives to prescription and other synthetic drugs to treat their illnesses. It wasn't long before acupuncture schools sprang up across the country. These days, most Westerners have heard of this and other Chinese arts, including tai chi and qigong, the therapeutic exercises that complement the medicine, but in the early '70s, these were new and exotic practices.

"With time and patience, the mulberry leaf becomes a silk gown."

—Chinese proverb

The Marriage of East and West

One of the great gifts of a global economy is that everyone can benefit from the best of what each culture has to offer. In China, Western medicine's technological applications are being used in the same hospitals that practice TCM. Likewise, TCM has presented itself to the Western world and is more welcome there every year. Estimates show that by the year 2000, approximately 2 billion people had taken advantage of what Chinese or Oriental medicine had to offer. The National Commission for Certification of Acupuncture and Oriental Medicine (NCCAOM) has offices in 38 American states, and their numbers continue to grow. In 2000, there were approximately 10,000 national-board-certified acupuncturists practicing in America.

These days, many medical doctors have incorporated elements of TCM into their practices, or have at least begun referring certain patients to TCM practitioners so they can explore the healing properties found in acupuncture and medicinal herbs. Some medical facilities have certified acupuncturists on their premises. And although American medical schools may not have the same syllabi as places that teach Chinese medicine, they are making strides. Stanford University has conducted joint studies with the National Cancer Institute and the College of Physicians and Surgeons at Columbia University and concluded that TCM is effective in regenerating organic functions and treating chronic disease. (Irritable bowel syndrome, if you hadn't noticed, is a chronic condition.) This is good news for those who feel better when an American institution of higher education gives a "new" medical treatment its stamp of approval.

Angela's Story, Age 32

After I found a doctor of Chinese medicine, the cramping and irregular bowels I had lived with for twelve years virtually went away. It was great because I never thought I'd be free of that excruciating pain.

Then, I went into labor with my first child. I couldn't believe it, but about two hours into labor, in the early stages, I heard myself say, "I know this pain! It's just like having IBS again!"

So now when people say that nothing comes close to the pain of labor, I say, "You've never had IBS."

Qi, Nature, and the Relationship of All Things

According to the ancient doctrines of Chinese healing, disease occurs because of an imbalance in the flow of Qi (pronounced "chee") within our bodies. This brings us to the first opportunity for you to free yourself from the tradition of Western thought and open your mind to concepts for which there are no direct English language translations. Simply put, Qi is the animating life force. It's energy. It's breath. It's whatever occupies something that reveals that there is life. But Qi is not only in our physical bodies; it's the vigor behind our thoughts, emotions, and spiritual lives. Plus, it defines nature, as well as permeates it.

In the human body, Qi flows in currents called meridians or channels (jing luo) and is responsible for five functions within the body, including:

- **Transforming** what we eat and drink into nourishing substances
- **Transporting** the nutrients to muscles and other body parts, as well as enabling the body to move and transport itself
- **Warming** the body
- **Protecting or defending** the body from external invaders (such as pathogens)
- **Containing or restraining** blood in the vessels, fluid in the bladder, organs in place, and so on

We carry about twenty types of Qi within our bodies, all of which are designed to protect and maintain human life. When everything is running smoothly, we are said to have Upright or Righteous Qi (zhen qi), which means we're healthy. When Qi is blocked, invaded by pathogens, or not running smoothly, we develop an illness, disease, or other physical or emotional imbalance.

A fundamental premise behind TCM is that human beings are part of nature—as much a part of it as the moon, ocean, trees, elements, and animals. Since Chinese medicine has been around so long, there are many different ways to describe this premise, but throughout history, the heart of the matter has remained the same. It involves five tenets:

🍃 As we are part of nature, we are subject to the same laws that govern nature and the universe. We are, essentially, a microcosm of the natural world around us, but since the same laws apply within as they do without, we can learn from nature and the universe about what is happening within our own bodies.

🍃 Living in harmony with the laws of the universe reaps a balanced life and good health.

🍃 Life is constantly transforming. Nothing is absolute except change.

🍃 Everything is related. There is order in the seemingly random design of nature, and that order is based on relationships between all things. To that end, good and bad are not absolute. They are relative.

🍃 People are not exempt from the relationships that balance nature. We are intrinsically connected to nature and the universe. Everything in the universe is a continuum of all other things. Our health is also product and reflection of this dynamic.

"To practice five things under all circumstances constitutes perfect virtue: these five are gravity, generosity of soul, sincerity, earnestness, and kindness."

—Confucius

Still, humans do play a unique role in nature because we occupy the space between heaven and earth, while also being dependent upon them both. Being healthy, or having Righteous Qi, is a product of when air Qi (that which flows from the heavens) and food Qi (that which sprouts from the earth) are one. The stuff from the heavens answers to our spiritual needs; the stuff from the earth answers to our physical needs. We cannot live without the life-sustaining qualities of both. Together they create both spiritual and physical balance, or health. This is the way of the Tao.

"He who lives in harmony with himself lives in harmony with the universe."

—Marcus Aurelius

When an imbalance (or illness) occurs, TCM instructs us to look at all aspects of our lives, not just the physical. We must view it with some altitude—from the perspective that we are dependent on both heaven and earth for our wellness. As such, we must refer to the vast array of influences and laws that support and characterize the balance of nature itself.

> "All these [Chinese] people are trying to retain their proper place in nature because their notion of health is that the body has to reflect the balances in nature. So, as the seasons change, people are supposed to be outside in the seasons, and when they're outside, they're supposed to feel their energy. When they feel their energy, they can become balanced, but if they don't feel their energy, then they fall out of balance, and they get sick."
>
> —Dr. David Eisenberg
> in Bill Moyers'
> *Healing and the Mind*

Yin and Yang: The Endless Circle

In TCM, yin and yang determine balance. Again, there's no English translation, but there are plenty of examples. Night is yin; day is yang. Winter and cold are yin; summer and heat are yang. Sitting still and going inward are yin. Running and shouting are yang. It's easy to reduce the meaning of yin and yang to that which is opposite. This may be so, but it's not the whole story.

Consider now that these aspects are different expressions of the same thing. Night and day are not opposites when you view our planet from outer space. Indeed, they are simply different shades and intensities of light reflecting off different sides of the same orb. Likewise, winter and summer are simply different expressions of the same natural phenomena of seasons. Shouting isn't only the opposite of meditating; it is also just another way of *being* from the same individual. Rather than reducing yin and yang to opposites, begin to see them as cycles within the whole.

"The power of the world always works in circles, and everything tries to be round. The sky is round, and I have heard that the earth is like a ball, and so are all the stars. The wind in its greatest power whirls; birds make their nests in circles, for theirs is the same religion as ours. The sun and moon, both round, come forth and go down again in a circle. Even the seasons form a great circle in their changing, and always come back again to where they were. The life of a person is a circle from childhood to adulthood, and so it is in everything where power moves."

—Black Elk

Yin and yang energies are both independent from each other and completely interdependent. There is always a little yin in every yang, and a little yang in every yin. Take a tree, for example. The big cottonwood that flourishes by the river reaching ever upward to the heavens, is yang. But quietly nestled within the tree are seeds, which are yin. The seeds themselves are incubating the next generation of trees within their tiny walls. Someday, the big cottonwood will cease growing and its yang energy will turn quiet, transforming into yin energy. At the same time, the seeds will fly to their new nesting grounds and suddenly burst forth with new life, full of yang energy, and become trees themselves. Inherent in this relationship is both independence and interdependence. One cannot flourish without the other. And in time, their cycles give way to the expression of the other. This is the great balance within life, and it's what's referred to as the Law of the Unity of Opposites.

There are yin and yang cycles within a day (sleep is yin; wakefulness is yang), within a year (dormancy during winter months is yin; activity during summer is yang), and within a lifetime (infancy is yin, childhood and young adulthood are yang, and the elderly years are yin again). It can make the cycles of your life easier to endure if you think in terms of yin and yang because you'll know that if there is overall balance, each energy will transform into the other at another stage of life.

"All human life has its seasons and cycles, and no one's personal chaos can be permanent. Winter, after all, gives way to spring and summer, though sometimes when branches stay dark and the earth cracks with ice, one thinks they will never come, that spring, and that summer, but they do, and always."

—Truman Capote

Female energy is considered yin, while male energy is considered yang. Don't panic: This doesn't mean that guys are supposed to do nothing but hunt bison and women are restricted to tending the fire and quieting the babies. The operative word here is *balance*. So, if you're career driven (yang), it would be wise to take some time out for stillness (yin). If you're a stay-at-home parent (yin), it would behoove you to go out on occasion and kick up your heels, or at least take a class (yang). Yin and yang energies play equally important roles within our lives, but it's up to us to balance how we play them out.

Life in the new millennium—just as it was 4,000 years ago—is a process of finding balance. Health is also process-oriented and always relative to something else within the universe in which we live. Western medicine may eye contradictions in this premise, but to the Chinese, all of the universe and its relationships are subjective and can only be interpreted within the context of its living subject. This means that when there is an imbalance, you must look from the inside out to determine the big picture and thus treatment, not just from the outside in.

Shen-jing is the Chinese term for doing this. Shen means waking consciousness, while jing means physical and material. Shen-jing pushes the current concept of a mind/body relationship a step further. It suggests that our health and well-being are also dependent on spiritual consciousness and the spiritual relationships between all things. By being wakeful in our consciousness, or spiritual life, we will also keep our physical bodies more in balance. This principle applies to our environment, as well. If we are not wakeful and conscious in how we interact with our planet, then we will create imbalances that will, in turn, affect our own health. It's a circle made up of endless relationships and interactions.

> "When you make the two one, and when you make the outside like the inside, and above like below; when you make the male and female as one, then you will enter the kingdom of God."
>
> —Gospel of Thomas

Blood, Balance, and the Impact of Climate

The Chinese attribute the qualities of yin and yang to parts of our spiritual and physical bodies. Qi is yang, while Blood is yin. Blood is not only the biological red plasma running through our veins, however. Blood is the balancing energy of Qi. British acupuncturist Francesca Diebschlag described it this way: "The movement of Qi is linear, from A to B. It's about creating new things, mastering new skills, conquering new territory. The movement of Blood is cyclic. It covers the same ground again and again, around and around on the same path, supporting and nourishing."

In essence, Blood is the inner self, while Qi is the outer self. But like the seed and the tree, they cannot survive without the other. Without the nutritive qualities within Blood, Qi wouldn't be able to do its job of protecting the life within its subject. And without the protection of yang energies, Blood would not be able to maintain its nurturing role. Blood also maintains Moisture in the body. Without it, life would be depleted.

The combination of Qi, Blood, and Moisture creates balance in the body. Blood governs the material form of the body, moisture governs the internal networks, and Qi governs the overall system. This relationship applies to both the larger and smaller systems in the body, such that if a lesser system is out of balance, it will impact the larger system, and vice versa. In essence, equilibrium is the balance of yin and yang throughout the body.

When an imbalance occurs, there is typically too much Qi, too little, or an uneven flow of it somewhere within the body. There are three reasons that Qi loses its balance:

1. **Internal pathogens**. Emotional energy lives within the body. If someone harbors resentment, it will affect an organ of the body—specifically the Liver—which in turn causes an imbalance of Qi. The intensity with which the resentment is experienced as well as the length of time it is harbored can affect the imbalance and how it is physically manifested.

2. **External pathogens**. Just like flu bugs or germs that Western medicine is so accustomed to, the Chinese do recognize that our bodies are invaded by outside forces. In this discipline, however, the invaders are associated with the properties of Mother Nature's weather report. The five external pathogens include:

- Wind—It can be gusty, as in spasmodic coughing attacks, or mild and dry, as expressed by chronic, constant, dry coughs. It can change course by starting out as a cold and ending up as the flu. Wind seeps into our bodies as often as it can, and because of that, it is considered to permeate more frequently than the other external pathogens. Wind causes a long list of health problems (fright, dizziness, tremors, headaches, strokes, skin sensitivity, and more), and it can kick up other pathogens such as Dampness, Dryness, Cold, and Heat. Symptoms can come and go quickly and leave you spent.

- Heat—It makes sense that Heat creates fevers and rashes, increases metabolism, activates circulation, and dilates blood vessels. But it is also the reason for inflammation, dry throat, constipation (aha!), agitation, welts, sores, boils, and more. It's also logical that when you suffer from an imbalance due to Heat, you crave cold foods and drink. But beware: Heat can exacerbate the effects of sugar, coffee, spicy foods (considered Heat producing), amphetamines, and alcohol, while also affecting the thyroid, adrenal glands, and the function of vitamin B.

- Cold—Shivering, colds, a repressed metabolism, and imbalances that show up as white or gray are products of Cold. Cold also contributes to skin problems and stress. When you have a poor diet, imbalances of Cold can result. Foods that are Cold can make symptoms of Cold worse. Antacids are considered Cold and are supposed to put out the Heat in the stomach (which is a problem because stomachs depend on digestive Fire to function properly). Cold medicines, antibiotics, aspirin, and antacids are Cold and upset digestion, which can weaken the overall digestive tract. People experiencing Cold tend to crave warm foods.

- Damp—Think swamp. Stagnant, heavy swamp. When you have too many fluids in your system, as in congestion, diarrhea (aha!), water retention, and swelling, or when you have dull pain, lethargy, or thick-headedness, you have been invaded by Damp. Dampness doesn't usually show up unaccompanied. It typically appears with Cold, Heat, or Wind, any combination of which can present a varied array of miserable symptoms. Dairy products, some fruits, starches, alcohol, and fatty foods should be avoided during times of Dampness.

- Dry—Everything from dehydration, brittle and flaking skin and nails, constipation (aha!), dry eyes, and loss of Blood (or Moisture) are the physical effects of Dryness. Ironically, long bouts of Dampness resulting in diarrhea can cause Dryness and constipation within the body. Excessive Dryness can invite other external pathogens to join forces and make things even worse.

3. **Trauma.** A broken bone, a severe laceration, or any kind of sudden trauma to the body causes Qi to center on the injury, thus interrupting the natural flow throughout the rest of the body. If the Qi remains fixed on the injury, then the rest of the body becomes depleted, which will eventually create more imbalances.

Even though much of TCM is complex, some of it is elegantly simple. As part of reinstating balance, the practitioner simply looks at the yin and yang qualities of the pathogens, then applies treatments that comprise opposite qualities. Symptoms created by Heat, for example, are treated with Cold properties. Where there is Dampness, the doctor would introduce elements of Dryness. When the flow of Qi is interrupted due to Trauma, the practitioner may apply acupuncture to redirect the flow. This follows the theory that the body has its own natural healing mechanism and tends toward homeostasis. The practitioner simply helps the body regain balance, at which point it will realign itself with health, or Righteous Qi, and life will continue with vigor.

Don't be misled, though. Treatment may be simple in some ways, but it refers to a complex system within the body and responds to a unique combination of pathogens and symptoms that the patient brings into the office. Since each patient is unique (even if symptoms are similar), each patient will have a unique treatment. To do that, the practitioner must explore both external and internal influences.

Internal Organs as Messengers of Health

The internal organs play an integral role in diagnosing imbalances and regenerating health. That vital role is why, in TCM, the organ names are always capitalized. Each organ contains either yin or yang energy and must carry out a specific function to help maintain balanced Qi. Naturally, the organs are dependent on each other for overall well-being, which is why they are referred to as the organ network, or shen. Shen is also governed by Qi. This perspective is a far cry from the exclusively biological one that Western medicine takes. Open your mind to the symbolic and organized relationship between the organs, and you may glean some insight into your own life situation. First, let's look at the yin/yang relationship of the organs.

Hollow organs (Gallbladder, Small Intestine, Stomach, Large Intestine, and Bladder) are considered yang and are busily transporting, digesting, containing, or eliminating. Solid organs (Liver, Heart, Spleen, Lung, and Kidney) are thought to store Essence, the highest form of Qi. When a yin organ is struck with disease, it is considered more severe than if an imbalance occurs in a yang organ.

Each organ network maintains a physiological job, but they also reflect spiritual, emotional, and mental aspects. Staying true to the nature of yin and yang, each organ is paired with another.

HEART AND SMALL INTESTINE

Heart. While the physical function of the Heart is to pulsate blood through the body, its spiritual job is to house shen, which is also called waking consciousness or the seat of consciousness (not only spiritual but physical alertness, as well). Because of that, the Heart is not solely yin, but rather encompasses both yin and yang. As such, it has the role of ruler or supreme commander and embodies both heaven and earth. It oversees order and prosperity and allows creativity, communication, and interaction. But it is dependent on nourishment from the Blood, or anxiety, despair, or insomnia may ensue. Other imbalances related to the Heart include anorexia, bad circulation, heart troubles, hypoglycemia, low blood pressure, manic depression, schizophrenia, and talkativeness. The primary emotion of the Heart is joy. But if joy is not balanced, if gratification and pleasure become the primary focus, Qi can be dispersed and can easily dissipate and turn joy into fright. Creating time for spiritual awareness helps harness joy and use it to maintain balanced Qi.

Small Intestine. Biologically, this organ discerns the nutrients in food and separates them from the waste. From the Small Intestine, fluids flow to the kidneys, while solids trot down the gastrointestinal (GI) tract to the large intestines. Metaphysically, the Small Intestine oversees the sorting out of relevant and irrelevant, the pure from the impure. The organ must be in balance to efficiently assimilate that which is nurturing and discard that which is unnecessary. San jiao is the transformation that occurs within the body between the entry of food and the exit of waste. Digestion and metabolism are governed by san jiao. (Digest that thought for a moment!)

LIVER AND GALLBLADDER

Liver. The Liver's job is to both store the Blood and make sure that it's distributed to all the places it needs to go so that Qi is evenly distributed throughout the body. Its spiritual job is to house hun, which is the ethereal soul or spirit. The Liver also governs emotions, leading the way to balanced Qi when the individual is self-aware. In the absence of such balance, or if emotions are blocked, then eruptions of anger, the primary emotion of the liver, can result. Other emotional manifestations include awkward social behavior, chronic tension, depression, erratic emotions, frustration, intense vacillation, and volatility. Physical disturbances include hemorrhoids, irritable bowel syndrome (aha!), migraines, poor circulation, premenstrual syndrome, ulcers, and unhealthy genitalia. Virtue, benevolence, flexibility, and kindness transcend imbalances of the Liver. Like the Blood it transports to the rest of the body, freeing emotional energy ensures good balance.

> "If you are patient in one moment of anger, you will escape a hundred days of sorrow."
>
> —Chinese proverb

Gallbladder. This organ stores and secretes bile that stimulates peristalsis, the natural contractions of the stomach and intestines that lead to defecation (aha!). The emotional function of the Gallbladder is to carry out what is just and correct with clarity of judgment. If in balance, the Gallbladder is responsible for making plans and turning fantasy into reality with its sharp analytical abilities. The Gallbladder also helps us recover after an emotional shock. If out of balance, we lose sight of the bigger picture, no longer have the vision to see things through, and are not as emotionally resilient.

SPLEEN AND STOMACH

Spleen. In Chinese medicine, the Spleen is far more significant an organ than in Western medicine. In TCM, it is responsible for supplying the nutrients that maintain Qi and Blood, which it governs, keeping us healthy and alive. After we eat, the Spleen oversees digestion and the subsequent assimilation of nutritional essence.

Ultimately, it transforms food (that which is not you) into generative energy (that which is you) in a process called hua. The Spleen rules metabolism and regulates and distributes Moisture—both critical functions for balanced Qi and Blood, as well as all other organs. The Spleen is the master of passages, transformation, and transmission. The spiritual charge of the Spleen is to house yi, or intellect and memory. When in balance, the Spleen creates coherency, meaning, purpose, stability, and the ability to cope with stress, engagement of ideas or thoughts, intention, and spontaneity. While faithfulness and reliability are its virtues, an imbalanced Spleen causes muddled thinking, obsession, and overthinking. Its primary emotion is worry. Physical manifestations of an imbalanced Spleen include arthritis, bloating, bruising, coldlike symptoms, dizziness, edema, fatigue, irritable bowel syndrome (aha!), lethargy, phlegm, scattered thinking, sore muscles, and becoming flabby, heavy, and worrisome.

Stomach. The job of the Stomach is to decompose food so that it can be sent to the Spleen for further refinement. The Stomach's motion pushes naturally downward, but if there is an imbalance and Qi moves upward through the Stomach, physical disturbances such as belching, hiccups, and regurgitation can occur. On the other hand, if there is too much downward push, the individual can experience diarrhea (aha!) and other lower bowel dysfunctions.

LUNG AND LARGE INTESTINE

Lung. It's nothing new to Westerners that breathing and respiration are a function of the Lung. But in TCM, breathing Qi into the body also regulates the body's rhythm, order, and homeostasis. Dispersing Moisture is also one of its tasks. The Lung governs the marriage of the inside world and the outside world, while also firmly setting limits and boundaries. It unites the essence of air Qi and the essence of food Qi. Lung energy enables us to live in the present with peace of mind (from the heavens) and physical vigor (from the earth). Spiritually, the Lung houses po, the corporeal soul of the physical body. While in balance, the Lung ensures that the physical boundaries of the body are intact, as represented by moist and malleable skin. The Lung also oversees wei qi, the ability of the body to adapt to the environment and protect itself from pathogens. When out of balance, physical symptoms of the Liver include asthma; dry skin; compromised immunity to colds, flus, and other infectious invaders; constipation (aha!); excessive sweating; headaches; loss of body hair; respiratory ailments; shortness of breath; and uncontrollable urination. The primary emotion associated with the Lung is sorrow. When the emotional energy is out of balance, one may feel controlled, detached, easily irritated, or shut down, and may avoid risk or passion. A balanced emotional life transforms sorrow into reverence (sorrow without pain) and honors each moment as unique and valuable.

Large Intestine. The Large Intestine receives the solid waste from the Small Intestine and has the final job of digestion and elimination. Metaphorically, the Large Intestine decides what needs to remain and what must be expelled, what's right and what's wrong, what's useful and what's not. When it is not in balance, our minds or our houses are cluttered, and we can't let go and make room for the new. There is a lack of clarity, a need to control, and a posture of rigid nonconformity. Physical manifestations include constipation (aha!), irritable bowel syndrome (aha!), rigid muscles, and a tight grip on opinions and possessions.

KIDNEY AND BLADDER

Kidney. Considered by the Chinese to be the organ that stores Qi and preserves what is essential, the Kidney itself is indeed essential to life. It is a double organ with a double function—to balance Fire and Water in the body. This means it must supply all other organs with both Moisture (yin) and Warmth (yang). Although primarily yin, the Kidney is also the only organ assigned properties of both yin and yang, and it is believed to be the root of yin and yang energy. Its spiritual job is to house zhi, or will and ambition. It is the organ that joins life and death, past and future, spiritual stability and endurance, imagination and visionary inspiration. It governs intellect, the instinct to survive, and our creativity. Its virtue is wisdom; its primary emotion is fear. When out of balance, fear can manifest as cynicism, paranoia, a preference for isolation or escape, and an expectation of the worst from life. When balanced, however, the Kidney is responsible for our power and skill. It oversees the reproductive organs, and as such, it makes sure that our family's physical and cultural codes are passed on to us and will be passed on to our children. The Kidney also oversees spiritual and physical growth and ensures that the fluids within the body are balanced. When there is a Kidney imbalance, physical expressions may include abdominal bloating, arthritis, chronically cold limbs, deafness, diarrhea (aha!), edema, joint deterioration, pain in the lower back and knees, phlegm, poor vision, premature ejaculation, prematurely gray hair, ringing in the ears, and senility. When in good balance, the Kidney provides us with balanced metabolism, clear thinking, energy, good sensory experiences, a healthy sex drive, steady and firm bowels (aha!), stamina, strong bones and teeth, and strong immune systems.

Bladder. Upon receiving fluid from the Kidney, the Bladder turns it into urine and eliminates it from the body. This completes the transformation and transportation of that which enters and that which must exit the body. It also regulates the vitality of the entire organism.

You may be feeling slightly overwhelmed by the many aspects that make up the science of traditional Chinese medicine. It can help to think of an orchestra and how each player works together to create the magical sounds of music. There are string, woodwind, percussion, and brass sections. There is a conductor and a song, and within the song there is melody, rhythm, and tempo, all of which contribute to the balance of the music.

Likewise, in an orchestra made up TCM, Qi would act as the conductor, while Blood and Moisture would be the melody, rhythm, and tempo. The instruments themselves would include the climate, or season section, the organ section, and the element section. (No, you don't know about that one, yet—but you will soon.) Meanwhile, keep in mind that yin and yang together are the harmonies that make the song work. So even if this does seem slightly daunting, hang in there; it's all going to come together soon so you can create a new theme song ("I feel good . . . like I knew that I would").

The Five Elements

There are five elements in TCM that represent energy and transformation. They are the same five elements known in the Western world, but again, by taking their meaning a step further—into the emotional, mental, and spiritual—you'll get the gist of what those ancient Chinese sages were up to.

Before illustrating what the elements represent, remember that TCM places humans deep within the web of nature. Including elements as part of what defines health and well-being links us to the environment and enables us to take the meaning of pathogens, climate, and organs to a deeper level. Using elements is also another way to show how each aspect of TCM is dependent on complex relationships within nature.

Each element is allied with a season, a climate, an organ, yin or yang, a sense, a body tissue, an emotion, a color, and a taste. It should be clear by now that if one of the elements is out of balance, there will be an impact not only on that which is allied with the particular element but also on the other elements and their affiliates, as well. What this boils down to, and all you really need to remember, is that *it's all related*. All of it. No isolating one thing from another here. In the most concrete terms, it means that if you break your arm, your back muscles (among other things) will be impacted, even though you didn't break the bones in your back. That's because how you walk, carry a bag of groceries, sleep, and breathe are all affected by the posture and weight-bearing demands of the rest of your body.

The five elements used in TCM are:

❦ Water
❦ Wood
❦ Fire
❦ Earth
❦ Metal

The following table diagrams the relationships between the elements and the other components you've learned about. To keep things simple, we're not including the related components of sense organs, body tissue, color, and taste.

The Five Elements and Their Relationships

WATER	WOOD	FIRE	EARTH	METAL
Kidney (yin)	Liver (yin)	Heart (yin)	Spleen (yin)	Lung (yin)
Bladder (yang)	Gallbladder (yang)	Small Intestine (yang)	Stomach (yang)	Large Intestine (yang)
Fear	Anger	Joy	Worry	Sorrow
Houses will and ambition (zhi)	Houses ethereal soul or spirit (hun)	Houses waking consciousness (shen)	Houses intellect and memory (yi)	Houses corporeal soul of the body (po)
Winter	Spring	Summer	Late summer	Autumn
Cold	Wind	Heat	Damp	Dryness

There is a specific relationship between the elements called the shen cycle (also called the nourishing cycle or mother/son cycle). This is defined by which element could be called the mother to the next. Water nourishes Wood, so Water would be the mother to Wood. Wood fuels Fire, Fire makes Earth, Earth yields Metal, and through condensation, Metal creates Water. Once again, we are in a never-ending cycle.

In the same but opposite way, there is the ko cycle (also known as the star cycle, regulating cycle, or grandmother/son cycle). It is illustrated by which element can consume the other. Water extinguishes Fire, Fire melts or tempers Metal, Metal cuts Wood, Wood can contain Earth, and Earth absorbs Water.

Both the shen cycle and the ko cycle are healthy and necessary for the balance of earth and nature. These cycles can be applied to our physical health, as well, when an imbalance occurs and treatment is necessary. For example, if there is too much Fire, treatment may call for properties associated with Water.

Take a deep breath. Remind yourself that you won't be tested on this. It's simply information that can help you establish a new way of looking at your own situation. What are you beginning to see?

"Today if you are not confused, you are just not thinking clearly."

—U. Peter

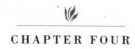

CHAPTER FOUR

Pattern Imbalances and Differential Diagnosis

Now that you've survived a crash course in traditional Chinese medicine (TCM), you're ready to seek out the best practitioner and volunteer to be a pincushion for an hour, right? Before making that first appointment, however, it may be helpful to review what the practitioner will likely ask, how she'll go about diagnosing your condition, and what your diagnosis may sound like. Clue: The Chinese don't have a term for irritable bowel syndrome. Rather, you'll probably be diagnosed with something that sounds like Spleen vacuity with Dampness encumbrance. To find out what that means to you, read on.

Western Disease versus Eastern Health

By now you know that there's an enormous difference between the worldviews of Western and Eastern medicine. It makes sense, then, that TCM would go about diagnosis and treatment in an entirely different manner. Indeed, if there were a single phrase to describe the premise behind Western medicine, it would be "find the disease and cure it with drugs." The phrase for Oriental medicine would be "practice holistic health and restore balance." Let's take a quick look at the practical realities of these differences.

SCENARIO 1: RALPH VISITS A MEDICAL DOCTOR FOR IBS

Ralph goes to his primary caregiver (who may have been assigned by his HMO and is someone he's never met) for an examination. The doctor asks general questions about his IBS, assesses the nature of his health profile, and prescribes drug X for his strongest symptom. If the doctor deduces that his IBS is mostly stress-related, he might prescribe an antidepressant. If he concludes that it's exacerbated by hyperacidity, he may suggest an over-the-counter antacid. And so on. Anyone else with the same symptoms would get the same or similar drugs. The drugs are prescribed based on the results of clinical studies where probably 50 percent or more of the subjects in the study respond relatively well to the medication.

If the doctor has time, he may ask about Ralph's diet and suggest more fiber intake. But when Ralph leaves the office, the doctor probably will not have asked how his insomnia is, if the pain in his knee has subsided, or if those chronic headaches have gone away. A quick scan of Ralph's chart alerts the doctor that he, or someone else, has prescribed sleeping pills and pain pills, but as far as he knows, they should work compatibly with this new drug he's prescribing. And chances are, since Ralph's there to see the doctor about his IBS, Ralph will neglect to tell the doctor that the pain pills make him feel nauseous.

Only after taking the new medication for several days will Ralph know if it reacts adversely with the other drugs he's taking. At that time, he can also determine whether he's part of the 50 percent of people for whom this new drug works or the 50 percent for whom it doesn't. If he does experience ill effects, it will be hard to know if it's due to contraindications between the drugs or just a side effect from the new one. His IBS symptoms may or may not be relieved. Meanwhile, Ralph is beginning to feel like a walking medicine cabinet, and he's grumpy because the insomnia is getting worse.

SCENARIO 2: RALPH VISITS A TCM PRACTITIONER FOR IBS

Ralph is asked to fill out the usual pile of paperwork with questions about family history and disease, and whether he smokes, drinks, or exercises—the same batch of questions he has been answering for years. But then he stumbles upon other questions that seem completely unrelated to the IBS. The questions include:

- What are the main health problems for which you are seeking treatment?
- List all other health problems you currently have.
- List any accidents you've had.
- Do you have chills/fever often? If so, at what time of day or night?
- Do you perspire heavily? If so, at what time of day or night?
- Do you experience pain or strangeness in your head or body?
- How often do you urinate? Is there pain?
- How often do you defecate? Is there pain?
- Do you have a good appetite?
- What foods do you crave?
- What's your favorite beverage?
- Do you have pain or swelling in your chest area?
- Do you have any gynecological problems?
- Do you have trouble with your ears or eyes?
- How well do you sleep?
- How strong is your sex drive?
- How do you feel about your spouse or significant other?
- How do you feel about your family?
- How do you feel about your diet?
- How do you feel about your sex life?
- How do you feel about yourself?
- How do you feel about work?

There are more. Puzzled, Ralph answers them and wonders if he's wasting his time.

When the practitioner examines Ralph, she asks questions about his IBS, but he notices the questions are different from the type asked by Western doctors. He's then instructed to stick out his tongue—and she takes what seems like a very, very long look at that. Then she takes Ralph's pulse in three different places. (Hmm . . . isn't there only one heartbeat beneath the skin?) She begins palpating his chest. Ralph wonders what his chest has to do with the pains in his abdomen. This is just the beginning of what turns out to be almost an hour-long exam that includes a host of questions.

The questions are not only about Ralph's IBS symptoms. This practitioner also wants to know all about his insomnia, knee problems, and those nagging headaches. Plus, she's interested in hearing about his stress level at work and home, too. By the time Ralph leaves the office, he feels thoroughly investigated and slightly bewildered at the depth with which the practitioner probed into his physical and emotional states.

In this scenario, Ralph will most likely take home some herbs or other supplements with funny-sounding names that are not only for his IBS but also to help with the headaches, knee pain, and insomnia. All of these are related, this practitioner would report. That never occurred to Ralph before, but according to TCM, they are all dysfunctions of the Spleen and Kidney—including the worry and fear he feels about his new boss. The herbs are supposed to help with everything.

The practitioner has checked to see if the herbs she's giving him will have contraindications with the prescription drugs Ralph is taking. She discovers they will not, nor will they present side effects of their own. Ralph may continue taking the prescription drugs if he desires, but the practitioner suggests that he may want to stop to see how the herbs work on their own. (If Ralph decides to quit taking his prescription drugs, he should notify his primary care doctor first.) She also recommends that he begin a stress-reduction program—meditation, yoga, or qigong. Ralph also has his first acupuncture appointment in a few days that will allegedly treat *all* of his health challenges.

"It's no longer a question of staying healthy. It's a question of finding a sickness you like."

—Jackie Mason

In both scenarios, the story doesn't end with the office visit. But what happens after the visits is as varied as the medical philosophies themselves. Hopefully, Ralph would get a positive change from either visit. But determining what's been effective and what's been treated marks the many differences between the two approaches. One approach is based on isolating the symptoms and treating them. The other considers Ralph's entire well-being, compares it to a model of health, determines how far he has deviated from health, and attempts to readjust his emotional and physical well-being to bring it back into balance.

Eight Guiding Principles and Patterns of Imbalance

As illustrated in Ralph's story, TCM takes into account every single imbalance you experience. The practitioner's ultimate job is to address everything you're up against and work with you until the balance of Qi has been established. She will ask about all the drugs and supplements you're taking, and she'll inquire about any side effects you've experienced. And she'll ask you some personal questions. In essence, she's evaluating your entire physical and emotional state to determine what's described as your *pattern of imbalance.*

Determining your pattern of imbalance takes time and requires a lot of information. The answers you provide will be linked to the Eight Pathological Factors, or Eight Guiding Principles. These comprise four pairs of two conditions, one yin and one yang. Linking your answers to these factors will enable the practitioner to ascertain the nature and location of your imbalance. The Eight Guiding Principles are:

Excess/Deficiency. How strong is the pathogen? How strong is your constitution? Is the nature of your problem from having too much of something (as in diarrhea) or too little (as in constipation)? Excess and deficiency usually refer to Qi, Moisture, and Blood. Acute illnesses are considered excessive, while chronic illnesses are thought to be deficient. Diseases of excess are often stronger than those of deficiency (or vacuity). IBS is considered a chronic condition, but your precise symptoms will determine whether your situation is one of excess or deficiency.

Interior/Exterior. Is the source of your imbalance internal, as represented in your deep visceral organs, bones, and emotional mechanisms? Or is it external, as shown on your skin, hair, and nails, or just under your skin at a muscle or joint? Deficiencies, emotions, and stagnation are usually related to internal imbalances. External imbalances include viruses, bacteria, and other atmospheric and environmental invaders. Some external pathogens may permeate the skin and bore into the interior of the body. Those are treated as internal pathogens even though they originated from the outside.

Cold/Heat. You may have cold extremities but a warm tummy. You may experience chronic colds. You may feel Cold about your work but warm and wonderful about your family. Cold is a condition caused by the lack of Heat, and it can manifest in one area of the body or spirit, but not in others. Some diseases are conditions of Cold, as are certain foods. Heat, meanwhile, produces conditions of excess Heat, and can also apply to your body, attitude, or the nature of the pathogen you are combating. You may feel a hot sensation when you need to poop. If this coincides with chronic loose stools or diarrhea, one of your diagnoses may be Damp Heat.

Damp/Dry. Usually related to bodily fluids, these conditions are either excessive in nature through Dampness or deficient in nature through Dryness. Phlegm, water retention, too much urine or feces—these all represent Dampness. Likewise, constipation, the inability to urinate, having no moisture in your sinuses or throat, or developing dry, flaky skin are all conditions of Dryness. IBS sufferers can fluctuate between experiencing Dampness (diarrhea) and Dryness (constipation). Being in either very humid or very dry climates can also cause or exacerbate these conditions.

Establishing the nature and location of your imbalance is one of several steps toward gaining an overall understanding of your health. But before making a final diagnosis, the practitioner will seek more information about you from your tongue and pulse.

Tracking Tongue Tales and Pondering the Pulse

Your tongue, according to TCM, speaks volumes about your health. The color, size, texture, and shape of your tongue reflects what's happening within your body, as well as in your emotional and spiritual life. A healthy tongue is bright pink and firm, with a smooth, thin white fur covering it. When you stick yours out, it will provide a map of sorts, guiding the practitioner to the location of your imbalances.

The back part of the tongue corresponds to the Kidney, the middle section to the Spleen, the front to the Lung and Heart, and the sides to the Liver. Indentations on the sides of the tongue may indicate weak digestion or a deficiency of Spleen Qi. A pale tongue can mean Qi Blood vacuity (deficiency). An overly red tongue suggests there's too much heat in your body, while purple says there's not enough heat. Red on the tip of the tongue speaks of an imbalance in the upper part of the torso, such as the Lungs or Heart. Spots on the side of the tongue indicate Liver Qi stagnation. If the tongue deviates to the left, it means one thing, while if it deviates to the right, it means another. A quiver says something about the strength of the Qi in your body, and so on.

The tongue fur may be the most revealing aspect for those with IBS, as it speaks to what's happening with the Qi in the Stomach, or the digestive Fire. Yellow fur indicates too much Heat in the stomach and can indicate pain and constipation. If you're bloated but have loose stools, it will probably show up as a thick white fur representing an excess of Cold and Dampness. A greasy, yellow fur (sounds appetizing, doesn't it?) in the middle of the tongue might suggest excess Heat and Dampness in the digestive centers. If the fur is dry or patchy, it can mean a deficiency of Moisture or Blood, as manifested in constipation.

Everyone knows, however, that if you eat some cottage cheese on the way to the doctor, you'll enter the office with a white, cheesy tongue. In the same vein, if you chow down on licorice or a strawberry lollipop, your tongue will absorb the color and texture of the sweets. Be mindful of this before visiting your practitioner. The natural condition of your tongue will tell the most accurate stories about your health.

Your pulse also provides insight into pattern imbalance. The speed, rate, rhythm, strength, and size of your pulse convey the qualities of your Qi, Blood, and Moisture in relation to the organ network.

There are three places on your wrist that correspond to the organ network. One area reads the attributes of the Heart and Lung. Another denotes the Stomach, Spleen, Gallbladder, and Liver. The third position tells about the Kidney, Bladder, Small Intestine, and Large Intestine. The practitioner will likely take your pulse at those three locations. The characteristics of the pulse in each area speak to the conditions of those specific organ networks.

The ancient Chinese scribes reported up to 32 pulse variations. In general, a slow pulse of under 60 beats per minute is associated with cool or Cold conditions. A pulse of over 80 beats per minute indicates Heat. A thinner pulse indicates fluid vacuity, while an exuberant pulse suggests an excess of fluid. If the pulse is superficial, it could mean the imbalance is more at the surface of your skin, or external. A deeper pulse means the pathogens are internal. If the relative strength of your pulse is weak, the pathogens have created deficiencies. A strong, fast pulse coincides with yang, while a thinner, weaker pulse does so with yin. Cold is yin, while Heat is yang.

The pulse can imply emotional imbalances, as well. According to some practitioners, people with IBS commonly have issues with frustration, worry, and the inability to let things go. Frustration is connected to the Liver, while worry and letting go are tied to the Spleen. These issues, too, will be unveiled through reading your pulse.

There are exceptions to all of these guidelines, however. A marathon runner's pulse, for example, may have fewer than 60 beats per minute and exhibit no conditions of Cold. The practitioner must factor in the constitution and lifestyle of each individual. (This is another reason practitioners ask questions that may seem more snoopy than pertinent. It's also a reason this expert will probably spend far more time with you than your HMO doc will.)

After examining your pulse, the practitioner may palpate your abdomen, chest, back, and acupuncture points along the meridians.

Tenderness at points along the meridians is usually a protective reaction to dysfunction and reveals more information about the imbalance within you. During phases of abdominal cramping associated with IBS, your colon may be extremely tender. Even a playful poke in the belly can incite rage from one who is vulnerable there. (You're probably well aware of that.) Likewise, you may have noticed your lap area can be either extremely hot or cold, depending on what's happening within your bowels. These are all telling signs to the trained eye and touch.

As the practitioner scans your tongue, feels your pulse, palpates your torso, and asks you questions, she will also examine you in other, more subtle ways. She'll take mental notes of the luster of your hair, the color of your nails, and the condition of your nail beds. She'll listen to the volume and strength of your voice and inhale the smell of your breath and body odor. She'll notice your walk, your posture, and how comfortable you seem with your body. She'll assess the texture and color of your complexion, and she'll notice whether it is uniform or blotchy. She'll home in on the shen (spirit) in your eyes and see if there are bags under them. Bags under your eyes could mean an imbalance of the Kidney—or that you had a good cry or a bad night's sleep. All these characteristics are viable resources and important ingredients for establishing your pattern of imbalance.

Differential Diagnosis

In Chinese medicine, it's practically unheard of to have a single diagnosis. Since everything is related, one imbalance typically leads to another. In Ralph's case, for instance, the headaches he experiences could be a result of toxicity in his colon from chronic constipation. The pain in his knees may be related to his worries about his new boss. We'll spare you the Chinese terms for all of Ralph's ailments, but this simply illustrates how rare it would be to leave the office of a TCM practitioner with one diagnosis.

What you'll get instead is referred to as a differential diagnosis. This is your unique blend of pattern imbalances, starting with the most severe and ending with the least imposing. Any combination of diagnoses is possible, but for someone whose primary problem is IBS with other, less-encroaching maladies, the primary diagnosis could be any one of the following:

❦ Retention of fluid due to Cold
❦ Damp Heat of the Gallbladder
❦ Heat in the Gallbladder
❦ Gallbladder Qi stagnation
❦ Damp Heat in the Large Intestine
❦ Large Intestine Qi deficiency
❦ Large Intestine Qi stagnation
❦ Stagnant Blood and Heat in the Large Intestine
❦ Liver depression Qi stagnation
❦ Liver Fire rising
❦ Cold and Damp in the Spleen
❦ Spleen Qi deficiency
❦ Retention of food in the Stomach
❦ Stomach Fire
❦ Stomach Qi deficiency
❦ Stomach yin deficiency

The diagnosis of Liver depression Qi stagnation describes alternating constipation and diarrhea along with bloating, an urge to defecate but difficulty doing so, plus other symptoms specific to certain manifestations of IBS. The Spleen Qi deficiency describes loose stools with a sense of bearing down pressure on the abdomen.

For those with chronic constipation and small, dry, hard stools, Liver Fire rising may be the diagnosis. Those who suffer from severe abdominal pains and vacillate between constipation and diarrhea could be told they have Heat in the Gallbladder. Excessive gas and belching with chronic stomach distension but regular bowels could be retention of food in the Stomach. This should give you an idea of the language you may hear and what it means when you are diagnosed by a TCM practitioner.

The examples here describe the simplest of symptoms. Most people with IBS experience a combination of many more complex symptoms. The variables of these symptoms add up to your unique differential diagnosis, and a good TCM practitioner will consider them all. Then, when preparing herbal formulas or preparing an acupuncture treatment, she will make sure to address all of your complaints.

Upon getting a diagnosis, if you're not sure what it relates to, ask the practitioner: Your Spleen? Stomach? Large Intestine? Then consider the emotions that are linked to that organ. Have you been experiencing them? Also, bear in mind that someone else with very similar physical symptoms may get an entirely different diagnosis. That's the beauty of this science: It will match up to your individual profile rather than stuffing your profile into a one-size-fits-most prescription bottle.

Feeling Out the Emotional Aspects of Dysfunction

Diagnosis is based on the answers to questions, an examination of your body, the nature of the external and internal pathogens, the Eight Guiding Principles, and how all of these components relate to the organ network. But emotional aspects come into play, as well. Migraine headaches may result from Spleen and Liver imbalances as experienced through worry and anger. As we've mentioned, those with IBS may have trouble letting go of things. Separating what's nutritious and what's not is the Spleen's job. If you can't discern between what serves you and what doesn't in your emotional and mental life, your Spleen can mirror that through abdominal cramping and other digestive disorders.

There is no single diagnosis for IBS because there is no single aspect to any one individual. But there are common threads among many people with IBS. Most typically, diagnosis involves dysfunction of the Spleen and Liver. As was discussed in Chapter Three, when things are going well regarding issues of the Spleen, the individual has the ability to cope with stress and is enveloped by a sense of meaning and coherency. When there's an imbalance of the Spleen, however, worry and overthinking result. When the Liver is in balance, the individual feels benevolent, flexible, and kind.

When the Liver is out of whack, the emotions of anger, depression, and frustration flare up.

In some cases, people experience physical deterioration first, which then leads to emotional imbalances. After all, it can be deeply disturbing if you have no control over when and where you poop. This can lead to anger or depression, which in turn can impact your Liver. Or you may be obsessed with how to do the grocery shopping—analyzing time and time again when to do it, which store has an accessible bathroom, and so on. This can throw off your Spleen. Once there is an imbalance in one organ, upsets will occur in other organs, surfacing as both physical and emotional disturbances.

Other times, it's the emotional imbalance that leads to the domino effect of physical problems. You may not be doing well at school or work, or your family life might be emotionally painful. You may feel a spiritual void, or you may be angry with God for a recent loss. Stresses—both large and small—can prompt physical illness. Repressing emotions, feeling ashamed, or thinking you're not worthy can all lead to physical complications. As you explore the path of wellness with a TCM practitioner, be prepared to take an honest look at your emotional and spiritual life and how it may relate to your physical symptoms.

You may believe everything in your life is going just fine. The emotional components of your situation may elude you. Take a step back, then, and look at the bigger picture. America is a culture in which competition is fierce. Material trappings have defined our worth and success. Money, to many, is God. Where do you fit into those values? Do you believe in them? Are you at peace with your financial situation? Do you have enough? Or are you striving for more and finding, on some very subtle level, that no matter how much you acquire, it's not enough?

Or are your underlying issues about beauty and youth? Do you consider yourself pretty or handsome enough? Does the constant barrage of media commercials make you think deep down inside that you need something more to be attractive? What about aging? Are you comfortable with growing older? Are you repulsed by older people? How do you feel about wrinkles? How comfortably do you sit with that extra weight on your midsection?

Cultural messages run deep. Even if you think you're happy or content, you may unconsciously want for more and ultimately feel empty inside. Those feelings can impact your health. Later in this book, we'll help you expand your awareness of how emotions play into your physical challenges and what you can do to constructively work with them.

Meanwhile, start to notice exactly what nonphysical cues set off an IBS attack. What were you feeling and thinking at the time? What kinds of stresses presented themselves? Did you feel good about yourself and others? Begin keeping a journal, and you may be surprised at what you find.

> "Pain and foolishness lead to great bliss and complete knowledge, for Eternal wisdom created nothing under the sun in vain."
>
> —Kahlil Gibran
> *Voice of the Poet*

The Risky Business of Self-Diagnosis

After reading this book, you may embrace TCM, read a few more books about it, do a little homework, and decide that you can become your own practitioner. We advise against that. Sure, excessive gas can be linked to the Large Intestine and Wind, but there's much more to it than that. Your gas may be a by-product of another, more pressing imbalance.

In China, it takes a minimum of four years of intense study to become qualified to treat people. A crash course taken by reading this and other books may inform you of the basics, but that doesn't mean you'll grasp the entire web of what's going on and be able to decide the appropriate treatment. In fact, trying to do that can be counterproductive. Purchasing premixed Chinese herbs based on self-diagnosis can actually worsen some of your symptoms, if you misunderstand the science. Keep reading, definitely take responsibility for helping yourself be healthy and happy, but by all means, use a professional for diagnosis and treatment. This stuff is dense—if you haven't noticed—and a trained professional is the most promising channel through which you'll find and maintain health and happiness.

> "It's not what we don't know that hurts us, it's what we know that ain't so."
>
> —Will Rogers

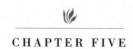

CHAPTER FIVE

Treating Imbalances with Acupuncture and Herbs

Adam's Story, Age 53

I've always been afraid of needles. When I was a kid, I used to throw up before getting a shot. As an adult, I've avoided going to the dentist, getting flu shots, and leaving the country because I just didn't want to get the vaccinations. My wife suffered from fibromyalgia for years, until she started working with a doctor of Chinese medicine. She loves getting acupuncture, and she urged me to try it to help with my IBS. The thought of it sent me in the other direction. But when I started seeing how much more energy she had and how much happier she was about everything, I finally decided I was being stubborn. The first time I went, I was very tense. My colon went crazy. The doctor was understanding and worked with me so that I didn't flinch when he inserted the needles. I didn't even feel it. And before long, I felt a subtle but very strong warm feeling take over. You can imagine my surprise when the doctor touched me saying our time was up. I fell asleep for the entire 45-minute session and didn't even know it!

Once a practitioner has determined your pattern of imbalance and differential diagnosis, he will treat you with acupuncture, herbs, massage, suggestions for dietary changes and exercises, or a combination of those things. Blending acupuncture with herbs is the most typical protocol and is considered comprehensive and effective treatment for just about any condition. Here's the lowdown on these two most common therapies.

Acupuncture: The TCM Tonic

If you've never had acupuncture before, you may conjure up images of sharp hypodermic needles thrust harshly into the delicate, baby-soft skin of your sensitive feet or other ever-so-vulnerable places. I mean, come on—most of us like the idea of being nibbled on the ear, but having someone stick a bunch of needles in it? No thank you.

Don't get your bowels in an uproar over this. Acupuncture can be as relaxing as a massage, as light as a tickle, and as potent as a nibbled ear—with even healthier rewards. So get over it. If you really want to know what a painless poop feels like, read on. Allow yourself to be frightened, but don't let that fear keep you from letting acupuncture change your life. Dive in, and prepare yourself for renewed energy and a healthier life. One last thing: There's a Chinese term for the unique and soporific feeling you may experience during or after an acupuncture treatment. It's called deqi (pronounced dah-chee). Translated to English (with a little poetic license), it means something like, "Oh-my-gosh-this-is-relaxing."

Here's how it works. If you recall, Qi courses through the body along fourteen main meridians, or channels. They run bilaterally (equally on each side of the body) in a vertical direction. Jing luo is the term for how Qi constantly flows along these channels, working in synch with the organ network and creating perfect, balanced health throughout your body. Unless, of course, it doesn't. And when it doesn't, the Qi is either blocked or imbalanced. The purpose behind acupuncture is to restore equilibrium to the physiological, psychological, emotional, and spiritual bodies that you occupy. (The makers of antacids don't share that mission statement.)

Although there are thousands of points along the 14 meridians, an acupuncturist usually targets about 300, 12 of which are primary points directly linked to one of each of the organs. If your imbalance is related to the Kidney, the practitioner will pinpoint (literally) the spots that correlate to the Kidney. If you also have a Liver imbalance, he'll go for the points associated with the Liver, as well.

Although there are approximately nine types of needles available for acupuncture, your practitioner will probably choose one of the six more commonly used needles. The needles are of different lengths, widths, and shapes at both the tips and the shafts. Rest assured that all of them are sterile and super thin—much finer than a strand of human hair. They're flexible, too, such that after they're inserted one-quarter to one-half inch deep, the acupuncturist may twist, turn, rotate, pluck, scrape, or tremble the needle according to which technique is appropriate. And there is a specific response that each technique summons, so trust that the acupuncturist isn't just experimenting or hoping to make you squirm. The truth is, you probably won't even feel any of those maneuvers.

Upon insertion, the needles may be positioned anywhere from 15 to 90 degrees relative to the surface of the skin. There will most likely be between one and fifteen needles used in the procedure. Most practitioners these days use (or should use) disposable needles to meet with biohazard regulations and guidelines. So if the fear of acquiring a transmittable disease is what's keeping you from trying acupuncture, you can relax. Choose to work only with a practitioner who uses disposable needles, and learning whether a certain practitioner does so is as easy as asking. In today's world, avoiding the risk of spreading disease is paramount, so put this concern to rest, and go for it!

Once the needles are inserted, amazing things happen. The Chinese say the needles simply restore balance. Western medicine likes to explain things through biological functions, though, so we'll give that point of view here, too. For reasons not yet understood, the needles stimulate nerves in the muscles just beneath the skin and send impulses through the spinal cord and up to the limbic system and thalamus of the brain. The pituitary gland, located in the mid-section of the brain, also receives the message. This stimulation triggers the release of a number of restorative chemicals from the brain, including the following:

Endorphins. These amino acids produced in the brain, pituitary gland, and spinal cord inhibit pain response, enhance mental clarity, and promote feelings of pleasure and relaxation by causing the release of dopamine.

Enkephalins. This endorphin specifically acts a neurotransmitter in the spinal cord and reduces feelings of pain.

Monoamines. These enzymes break down the pain-reducing effects of serotonin and dopamine.

Serotonin. This amino-neurotransmitter dampens the effects of pain.

Vasodilators. These dilate blood vessels and increase blood flow and circulation.

> "Because certain acupuncture points increase serotonin levels, the result is often a generalized decrease in the stress response. Most often, this is a welcome side effect of an acupuncture treatment for some other problem (such as backache or joint pain). Recently, a patient told me that since starting acupuncture treatments with me for a chronic lower backache, she has gotten rid of the constipation that has plagued her for 20 years. This reduction of stress-related problems is typical of acupuncture patients."
>
> —Kenneth Giuffre, M.D.
> *The Care and Feeding*
> *of Your Brain*

Acupuncture treatments can last for two minutes or for up to an hour, depending on the patient's needs. As was true with Adam, you may feel gentle warmth that puts you to sleep, a slight tingling sensation, or nothing at all. Usually, people feel extremely relaxed after a treatment, and many find it easy to nap afterwards. We've never heard of anyone running from the office screaming in pain and vowing never to return. On the contrary, many people look forward to their next session. This may occur biweekly, weekly, bimonthly, or anything in between—depending on your unique needs.

There are several types of acupuncture available, so don't be surprised if your practitioner suggests one of these techniques:

Electro-acupuncture. This technique is far more popular in China than America. Most commonly administered for pain relief, the practitioner applies a low electrical impulse through the needle. Higher frequencies are typically used for easing pain related to surgical procedures, while lower frequencies work for low-grade pain.

Auriculotherapy. Also known as ear acupuncture, many American practitioners rely on this treatment. Ears are loaded with nerves and blood, thus supporting the notion that they are well connected to the rest of the body and the organ network.

Moxibustion. With this technique, a practitioner applies heat to the acupuncture point by burning an herb (usually mugwort) at the site. Acupuncture and moxibustion are complementary and are often used together.

Cupping. In this treatment, acupuncture points are stimulated by applying suction through a vacuum created by a wood, metal, or glass device.

Acupressure. You may already be familiar with this technique. It's based on the same principles as acupuncture and in fact is performed in the same manner—only without needles. Also known as reflexology or Zone Therapy, you can invigorate your own health by using your fingers and stimulating specific points on the soles of your feet or ankles.(Many books are available to help you learn about performing this technique on yourself.) Professionals may also use an instrument with a hard, ball-shaped head for stimulation. Acupressure can be very enjoyable and relaxing, but using needles goes deeper with the healing process, giving you faster, more tangible results.

Eleanor's Story, Age 36

My mother had ulcerated colitis most of her life. There's a 20 percent chance that children will get the condition if one of their parents has it. I was the lucky one.

After thirteen years of taking a series of intravenous drugs to help with it, I was told there was no cure. These were very difficult times. Things got even worse after my mother was in a car accident. She was in terrible pain and was so tired of taking drugs for the colitis that she couldn't bear the idea of more pills on top of what she was already popping. A nurse suggested she try acupuncture to relieve the pain.

Within weeks, she was up and running without any more pain in her body. She liked the way she felt, so she continued with the treatments. Then she called me one day and told me her symptoms of colitis had vanished. She couldn't say for sure that the acupuncture had done it, but she admitted that she hadn't had any improvements whatsoever prior to having the acupuncture.

After my first acupuncture treatment, I felt slight improvement. After four sessions, my bowels returned to normal, the pain stopped, and I began to think I might live a normal, drug-free life. Now, three years later, I have no signs of colitis. I told my doctor about it, and he suggested that it was all in my mind and said that I should consider having a colostomy. I laughed. I'm still laughing.

ACUPUNCTURE AND IBS

Inserting needles in your skin to restore good health may seem like hocus-pocus to you, but it has withstood the test of time (the first written references appear in the *Yellow Emperor's Classic* by Huang Ti, composed thousands of years ago), and it is now creating quite the stir in Western medical circles. That's because studies conducted around the globe are confirming the remarkable health benefits of acupuncture and are finally offering the biological rationale that Western medicine depends on to validate procedures.

There haven't been many studies conducted regarding the benefits of acupuncture on IBS, although the Chinese have been successfully treating gastrointestinal disturbances for thousands of years. It's difficult to fit the complex, interrelated philosophy of Chinese medicine into the paradigm of Western medicine's

〜

The National Institutes of Health (NIH)
Endorses Acupuncture

In November of 1997, a panel of health experts gathered under the auspices of the NIH and agreed that acupuncture is a worthwhile treatment for a variety of different health conditions. The press release they distributed revealed:

"A consensus panel convened by the National Institutes of Health (NIH) today concluded there is clear evidence that needle acupuncture treatment is effective for postoperative and chemotherapy nausea and vomiting, nausea of pregnancy, and postoperative dental pain.

"The 12-member panel also concluded in their consensus statement that there are a number of other pain-related conditions for which acupuncture may be effective as an adjunct therapy, an acceptable alternative, or as part of a comprehensive treatment program. . . . These conditions include but are not limited to addiction, stroke rehabilitation, headache, menstrual cramps, tennis elbow, fibromyalgia (general muscle pain), low back pain, carpal tunnel syndrome, and asthma . . . .

". . . Adverse side effects of acupuncture are extremely low and often lower than conventional treatments. However, the panel noted that adverse side effects have occurred on rare occasions. They recommended that patients be fully informed of their treatment options, expected prognosis, relative risk, and safety practices to minimize the risks prior to undergoing acupuncture treatment. Because many individuals seek health care treatment from both acupuncturists and physicians, the consensus panel advocated a strengthening of communications between these health care provider groups to maximize the possibility that important medical problems are not overlooked. The panel additionally encouraged broader public access to acupuncture treatment by urging insurance companies, Federal and state health insurance programs including Medicare and Medicaid, and other third party payers to expand their coverage to include appropriate acupuncture treatments. Doing so, the panel stated, would help remove the financial barriers to access to these services. . . ."

"controlled studies." Even so, one study performed in England back in 1977 and published in *Hepato-Gastroenterology* claimed that "patients experienced a significant improvement in overall wellbeing . . . and showed a significant improvement in symptoms of bloating." The subjects had on average four to six visits to the acupuncturist over a period of twenty-eight days. Sixteen points were stimulated, and sessions lasted for less than two minutes. The longer the patient had been suffering from IBS, the more treatments were necessary.

Another study published in 1995 in *The British Medical Journal* indicated that specific acupuncture points are effective for normalizing various gastric disturbances since those points "affect motility and gastric secretion by stimulating peripheral nerve endings and releasing beneficial chemicals." They also learned that specific points are sedating points, and since many IBS patients have a "raised element of stress or anxiety," stimulating these points can also prove beneficial.

In plain English, that simply means that the practitioner will very likely target points associated with your Spleen and Liver. Secondarily, they may also choose points associated with the Large Intestine, Stomach, Bladder, and Gallbladder. Depending on your unique pattern imbalances, the acupuncturist will probably choose between one and nine needles for treatment.

📓

Most Medical Doctors Believe Acupuncture Works

According to a study published in the November 1998 issue of *The Archives of Internal Medicine* and conducted by the Stanford Center for Research in Disease Prevention, 51 percent of physicians surveyed believe in the efficacy of acupuncture. Of those, 43 percent actually refer their patients to an acupuncturist. Acupuncturists receive a higher rate of physician referral than any other method of alternative health care.

Bear in mind, however, that treatment from different acupuncturists for the same symptoms may vary. This is because each doctor may have a slightly altered interpretation of your patterns and will treat them according to what she believes is best.

Later in the book, we'll give tips on how to find a qualified acupuncturist in your area and what kinds of questions to ask. You may start your search by asking around—medical professionals, friends, family, and business associates are all good resources for this information. Word of mouth provides the best advertising for a good practitioner.

Before undergoing an acupuncture treatment, be sure to inform the practitioner if you are:

Pregnant. Some points will stimulate uterine contractions, and unless you're about ten months pregnant, that's not something to promote.

Taking anticoagulant drugs. Even these tiny needles can cause bleeding, so discuss the procedure with your medical doctor and the acupuncturist.

Living with a pacemaker. If you have a pacemaker, electro-acupuncture can interfere. Always let your TCM practitioner know that you have a pacemaker before beginning any new treatment.

Diabetic. This isn't a problem that would prevent you from receiving acupuncture, but it's something every health practitioner should know before administering treatment.

Andrea's Story, Age 32

I've had chronic back pain since I slipped a disc when I was 14 years old. Not long after that happened, I started to have bouts of bad constipation—sometimes for up to a week at a time. The constipation would be followed by days of diarrhea. I never went to a doctor for the troubles with my bowels; I just figured I had a sensitive system. But I went to plenty of doctors about my back. When someone suggested I have surgery to relieve the pain in my back, I decided to try a chiropractor.

Working with the chiropractor did a lot to help with my back. Eventually, I told him about my problems with going to the bathroom, and he put me on a new diet and some enzymes. It helped reduce the extremes, but it didn't get me completely regular. Finally, after about six months of working together, we came to an impasse. My back was a lot better, but not as good as we had both hoped. My bowels were better, but not great. The chiropractor then said he had done everything he could for me and advised me to try acupuncture.

I went to a woman who is pretty well known in my community for successfully relieving pain through acupuncture treatments. I thought she'd be all mellow because that's the stereotype of a Chinese doctor, but I've never met anyone with so much energy. The first time I saw her, I thought, "If only I could bottle up that energy and take it home."

I went to her expressly for my back pains, but she asked me about my digestive system, so I told her. It didn't take many sessions, maybe three, for the pain in my back to be completely relieved. But what amazed me was the improvement I experienced in my bowels. I wasn't expecting that. I went to her a total of about six times, and by the end, my bowels were pretty much normal every day. I still go to the acupuncturist about every three months, just for a tune up, but I'm living now for the first time with what must be "healthy regularity." The other thing that surprised me was that when I got my bowels in order, I had energy to spare.

Herbs: Nature's Medicine

Throughout history, nature has served as humanity's medicine cabinet. Only for the last 100 years or so—a mere blip in the timeline of humankind—has herbal medicine been considered "adjunct" therapy to mainstream medicine. Indeed, for thousands of years, mainstream medicine was literally rooted in the soil, and it sprouted as various herbs and plants that were effectively used for every ailment under the sun. Since Chinese medicine documents the oldest recorded herbal treatment, it could be considered the grandfather of the science.

We've already explained why America's current health care system chooses not to take the herbal path (you can't make a mint on plants because they can't be patented). But even the big pharmaceutical companies rely on plants to provide insight into healing properties. Ma huang is a great example. Five thousand years ago, the Chinese discovered that this herb promoted sweating and did wonders for the common cold, asthma, and other respiratory ailments. Many moons later, in 1924, the Chinese isolated ephedrine from the ma huang plant as the specific healing agent that did the trick. The American pharmaceutical companies immediately got busy and made a synthetic version of ephedrine. You'll find it in the myriad over-the-counter cold medicines available to you. Look at the ingredients of whatever cold medicine you have in your medicine cabinet; in just about every one, you'll see psuedoephedrine—the copycat of nature's organic solution. Moral of the story: If corporate America's top-paid scientists are creating chemicals that mimic the properties found in herbs, you can bet that the herbs themselves are good medicine—and mostly without the side effects the "pseudoversions" produce.

Remember Shen Nung? He was that really smart Chinese doctor that, more or less, came up with the idea of TCM. He also tested tens of thousands of plants, examined their medicinal properties, and discerned which one—or ones—worked with specific pattern imbalances to restore the balance of Qi. His blueprint of herbal therapies has been refined and perfected over thousands of years, and these days it comprises sophisticated and complex formulas that treat imbalances. The herbal pharmacists have also taken care to create the safest blends, so even though these herbal remedies are mighty powerful, they are usually free of side effects.

You may already use some herbs in your life, such as St.-John's-wort for depression or valerian for insomnia. It's rare to find someone in today's world who doesn't take advantage of herbal remedies. But those are single-plant remedies. When you are given a Chinese herbal formula, you will be taking a complex combination of herbs all designed to balance your unique differential diagnosis. According to an article published in *Pharmacology and Therapeutics,* the herbal formulas found in Chinese medicine are made up of as many as twenty different herbs, and each medicine is customized to a single patient.

Because of their complex nature, Chinese formulas are difficult for Western medicine to study through clinical trials. In essence, controlled studies depend on single-chemical entities so researchers can isolate which chemical property is having which effect. Meaning, when you take straight St.-John's-wort, studies are able to show which chemicals in the plant are specifically effective for relieving depression. You can't do that with Chinese herbs because most formulas rely on a *combination* of herbs for effect.

Attempts are being made by some advocates of TCM to assist Western researchers in creating new paradigms for studying Chinese formulas so they will be taken more seriously. Robert Yuan is one such researcher who has investigated studies of TCM as it is used to treat IBS and other chronic diseases. His review was published in *Pharmacology and Therapeutics* in May 2000. In it, he says, "we show how TCMs differ from therapeutics based on single-chemical entities, and outline how modern scientific and clinical procedures need to be adapted for the study of such herbal preparations. The studies cited. . . . show that when properly done, modern techniques can provide valuable information for the validation of specific TCMs, particularly in the prevention and treatment of chronic diseases."

The theory behind how herbs work is that when two or more plants are combined, several different dynamics, or characteristics, can result:

- 🌿 **Mutual accentuation.** When two compounds (or sets of compounds) with similar activities are combined, a stronger effect will result.
- 🌿 **Mutual enhancement.** When two compounds (or sets of compounds) with different activities are combined, they result in the enhancement of one by the other.
- 🌿 **Mutual counteraction.** When two compounds (or sets of compounds) are combined, the toxicity or side effects of one compound is reduced by the other.
- 🌿 **Mutual suppression.** When two compounds (or sets of compounds) are combined, each one can reduce the side effects of the other.

⚘ **Mutual antagonism.** When two compounds (or sets of compounds) are combined, each minimizes or neutralizes the activity of the other.

⚘ **Mutual incompatibility.** Neither compound (or set of compounds) is toxic, but when combined, it results in toxicity or side effects.

The article then explains that in Chinese herbal formulas, the principle ingredient is "a substance that provides the main therapeutic thrust. The second ingredient enhances or assists the therapeutic thrust of the first." The rest of the ingredients:

⚘ Treat other, lesser symptoms
⚘ Counteract the toxicity of the primary herbs
⚘ Guide the medicine to the proper organ
⚘ Exert a harmonizing effect

Ironically, technology isn't yet equipped to break down such multichemical formulas in a way that Western medicine can comprehend and categorize them. Nor are we able to understand how the combinations of these herbs can do what they do collectively. Rather than defer to thousands of years of successful treatment as proof of their validity, Western science continues its attempt to fit Chinese herbal combinations into clinical studies to prove their worth. Perhaps someday there will be a method in which allopathic doctors can justify, embrace, and even advocate using these mysterious and powerful combinations. Until then, I'm happy to ward off symptoms of any description with the same herbs that Buddha may have used. If I'm lucky, I'll be wiser for it!

Rita's Story, Age 30

At first I was told that I had IBS, but after time—and lots of blood in my stool—the doctor rediagnosed me with ulcerative colitis. It wasn't easy for me to believe that taking herbs and doing acupuncture could help with my condition. I had tried chemotherapy and so many strong prescription drugs, and they didn't do anything. How was I supposed to believe that plants and needles could help me?

Out of sheer desperation, I did a series of treatments and took specific herbs that my doctor of Chinese medicine said would help. He said it would take about four months for any sign of improvement, but I felt a difference after my first treatment. Two months later, there was no more blood in my stools and I began to feel good. It's been about a year, and I've weaned myself off all medications. I feel as though I was set free!

HERBAL TREATMENT FOR IBS

The Aussies are known for being a bold lot, and back in 1996 a group of medical professionals headed by Dr. Alan Bensoussan decided to broach the complex world of Chinese herbal formulas in a scientific manner. They conducted a year-long, randomized, double-blind, placebo-controlled trial in which the University of Sydney combined its efforts with two local teaching hospitals and five private practices to see just how beneficial Chinese herbs could be for treating IBS. *The Journal of the American Medical Association* (JAMA) published the study and its conclusions in November 1998.

One hundred and sixteen people who fulfilled the Rome criteria for having IBS volunteered for the study. A Chinese herbalist was invited to participate in the study, and he, too, diagnosed the subjects according to the tenets of TCM. Subjects ranged from 18 to 75 years old, and both genders participated about equally. Several different doctors and herbalists evaluated each person's unique etiology prior to treatment.

The group was divided into three smaller subgroups. Forty-three people were given a generic Chinese formula thought to regulate and strengthen bowel function. The second group of thirty-eight people took formulas based on eighty-one different herbs that the Chinese herbalist created specifically for each individual's profile. The third group of thirty-five people took a placebo.

All pills were given in capsule form and were made so that no one could tell the difference between the generic herbal remedy, the individual treatment remedies, and the placebos. Both the subjects of the study and those who distributed the pills were unaware of which group each subject occupied and what each subject was taking.

Everyone took five capsules three times a day for a 16-week period. The subjects were not asked to make any changes in lifestyle, diet, or exercise patterns. They were told to continue eating their usual diet and avoid those foods they thought worsened symptoms.

Each person was evaluated by doctors and herbalists 8 weeks after the study began, and then again at 16 weeks, when treatment was complete. A total of seventeen patients left the study for various reasons. At the end of the study, 44 percent of those who took the generic herbs said their symptoms had improved. M.D.'s who examined those patients cited a 59 percent improvement in the individuals in that group. Meanwhile, 42 percent of those taking individual herbal treatments said things were better, while doctor evaluations confirmed improvement among 40 percent. Among those who took placebos, 22 percent said their condition was better, while the doctors said 19 percent had actually improved. Of the patients who experienced a positive change, all claimed that IBS caused less interference in their lives while on the herbs and placebos.

Nearly four months after completing the study, 75 percent of those who had been taking the individual herbal formulas reported that they still felt improvement, compared to only 63 percent of those who had taken the generic herbs and 32 percent of those who had taken the placebo. The author of the study concluded:

> ". . . *Chinese herbal formulations may offer symptom improvement on some patients with IBS. In this randomized, double-blinded, placebo-controlled trial, Chinese Herbal Medicine (CHM) was shown to be effective in the management of IBS. Patients receiving the standard CHM formulation fared best during the course of treatment, while patients receiving the individualized treatments found that the benefit gained lasted beyond the treatment period. Although not all patients responded to this therapy, our findings support the consideration of further investigation of Chinese herbal medicine as a treatment option for IBS.*"

Authors of the review concur that administering a generic formula doesn't live up to the fundamental principles of TCM and that individual treatments are preferred. They also stressed that while undergoing herbal treatments, patients should be monitored at specific intervals so appropriate adjustments can be made.

Generic versus Custom-Blended Herbs

Although individual formulas are best for treating any condition, the generic herbal formula used in the Sydney study had the greatest effect on patients who took herbs during the sixteen-week treatment period. The standard formula was a combination of twenty different herbs combined in the percentages noted below.

Note: Individuals should never try to create their own combinations of herbs, but may find it useful to take this list to their practitioner.

CHINESE NAME	PERCENT POWDERED HERB
Yin Chen	13%
Bai Zhu	9%
Dang Shen	7%
Yi Yi Ren	7%
Wu Wei Zi	7%
Zhi Gan Cao	4.5%
Huang Bai	4.5%
Che Qian Zi	4.5%
Fu Ling	4.5%
Qin Pi	4.5%
Pao Jiang	4.5%
Hou Po	4.5%
Chai Hu	4.5%
Huo Xiang	4.5%
Fang Feng	3%
Chen Pi	3%
Bai Shao	3%
Mu Xian	3%
Huang Lian	3%
Bai Zhi	2%

❧

The Myth of the Magic Bullet

Hungry? Pop something in the microwave. Headache? Take an aspirin. Bored? Turn on the tube and flip through seventy-eight channels with the remote control. Unhappy? Have a margarita. Yellow light when you're in a hurry? Gun it.

Most things that annoy us during the course of the day can be diminished or eliminated—albeit temporarily, and sometimes at the expense of our health—within minutes, if not seconds. That's what we're used to, and that's what we expect. It's called instant gratification, and boy, when we don't get it, we get irritated.

Our attitude toward health care and medicine is no different. If we're sick, we take a prescription drug and expect to be better by tomorrow or the next day at the latest. Even with chronic conditions like IBS, we still look for the quick fix—even if we know it's only temporary. Better now and temporary than later and forever. Right?

Not according to Chinese medicine. Not according to real life. According to real life, the magic bullet doesn't really exist. Sorry.

But with time and patience (two things that are terribly underrated today), acupuncture and herbs can be highly effective in restoring your vitality and health. The changes you enjoy will unfold incrementally, as most lasting changes do. It takes time for your body to realign. It takes time to work out the emotional issues that relate to your physical limitations. It takes time to unwind, relax, and retrain yourself to think and behave, to prepare good food, to exercise, to meditate, to love someone for a lifetime. It all takes time. The good news is that just like everyone else who has turned his or her life around, you, too, have twenty-four hours in each day. It's just a matter of how you choose to spend them.

You've probably been living with IBS for a while. Give yourself a while to get better. Relax into it. You're not going anywhere. But if you stick with TCM, over time, your symptoms will.

As the first formal study to document how Chinese herbal medicine can treat symptoms of irritable bowel syndrome, this may open the door for other clinical trials that will eventually validate Chinese herbs in the minds of Western doctors. Until then (and don't hold your breath—it will take many years) we urge you not to self-diagnose and treat your condition with generic formulas. If high-paid researchers can't figure out how and why these herbs work, chances are you won't be able to, either. Instead, ally yourself with a professional herbalist or TCM practitioner, and reap the benefits of their expertise.

"Everything has been figured out except how to live."

—Jean-Paul Sartre

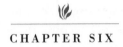

CHAPTER SIX

Finding a Qualified TCM Practitioner

Greta's Story, Age 28

My father was a prominent cardiologist in Boston, and I grew up believing that what doctors said was gospel. When I started showing signs of a spastic colon as an adolescent, Dad consulted with his colleagues and put me on prescription drugs. I don't know what they were—I didn't bother to ask, as I believed without hesitation that he knew what was best for me. Although the painful symptoms of my condition were relieved, I constantly fluctuated between constipation and diarrhea. I didn't care, as long as the pain was kept at bay.

Over time, though, I experienced bouts of dizziness, excessive dry mouth, and blurred vision. Dad knew it was probably from the drugs, so he took me off what I had been taking and put me on something else. Those side effects subsided, but I found myself bloated and fighting constipation on a regular basis. Losing faith in my Dad's choices, I secretly stopped taking the drugs. By that time, I was a junior in high school and becoming more conscious of how I looked. A bloated tummy wasn't on the list of things I wanted.

When I abandoned the drugs, constipation gave way to diarrhea, and then the pains came back. I was very depressed and finally told Dad what was going on. My mother had a friend with chronic fatigue who had gone to an acupuncturist who successfully treated her. When I heard about this, I was excited about trying something else. Reluctantly, Dad agreed to let me go, but I know he didn't tell his friends.

The acupuncturist was great. After one session with me, he put me on some Chinese herbs, suggested I eat "cleaner" foods (rather than the junk food I had been consuming), recommended stress-reducing techniques, and gave me acupuncture twice a month for about four months. By the time I graduated from high school, I was off prescription drugs, eating a healthy diet, and had figured out what foods and conditions spurred the painful cramps and bowel irregularities. It was a wonderful personal transformation for me to go from passively taking pills and hoping they would make me well to actively being aware of and involved in my habits, emotions, and body to be healthy.

Now, ten years later, I still practice good eating habits, I am addicted to yoga, and I keep myself as stress-free as I can. I don't mind having a sensitive colon anymore; I figure it's my body's way of keeping my habits in check. My Dad still doesn't understand why or how acupuncture works, but seeing the changes in my condition has helped open his mind to the fact that there is more to good health than writing a prescription.

Locating a good TCM practitioner is a similar process to finding a trustworthy medical doctor. It takes research, a few telephone calls, and firing off a series of questions to the most likely candidates. Then, compare what you want out of your experience with what each practitioner has to offer. Pretty simple stuff, but there are a few guidelines that can ensure that you are working with a well-educated and ethical acupuncturist.

Education and Licensing

Most practitioners of TCM will be skilled in both acupuncture and the art of understanding and combining the complex herbal formulas that make up the traditional Chinese pharmacy that is the basis of traditional Chinese medicine. In America, the only agency that monitors herbs is the Food and Drug Administration (FDA), and it is only slightly involved. It oversees label claims so that food and herbal supplements cannot claim to prevent, treat, or cure any disease or serious symptom of disease. It is also the entity that tests for contamination and takes action in the event that contaminated herbs are being sold. There are no educational requirements for working with and distributing herbs, although there are organizations that promote the safety and efficacy of "prescribing" them. California is the only state that requires practitioners to take exams in both acupuncture and herbology in order to distribute herbs for medical purposes and be considered a doctor of TCM.

The TCM practitioners you'll encounter are most likely to be licensed acupuncturists (L. Ac.) and diplomates of acupuncture (Dipl. Ac.), rather than doctors of Oriental medicine (D.O.M. or O.M.D.). There aren't many states that allow the title of doctor even for those practitioners trained in China who have earned a doctorate. There are a few programs throughout America that offer a master's in traditional Oriental medicine (M.T.O.M.), but it's impossible to say whether the individual with a doctorate or a master's has any greater knowledge than someone with a state license. Having a master's and doctorate does not in and of itself grant the right to practice, nor does it represent certification. That's because there are no standards or consistent rules in American-run schools with a master's program in TCM. So, you may find someone with a master's who has more schooling, but he is not necessarily more equipped than someone with a state license.

Each school assigns its own definitions to different levels of education, just as each state determines its own licensing requirements. Hence titles and licensing can mean very different things from school to school or state to state. The most important aspect of your search for a good acupuncturist is that he or she be licensed, and a license can only be granted through the state in which the practice is located.

There are no licensed acupuncturists from the states of Alabama, Georgia, Idaho, Indiana, Kentucky, Nebraska, Ohio, Oklahoma, Tennessee, and Wyoming because those states don't recognize or regulate the field of acupuncture. If you live in one of those states, however, you may well find someone who is practicing there but is licensed by a different state. This is tolerated in most states, even though it's not actually legal. At least not yet. Legislation has been introduced in each of those states to legalize and recognize acupuncture and to open the door for licensure of acupuncturists who live there.

In the states that do recognize and regulate acupuncture, each one has its own unique educational requirements. In California, for example, the nearly 5,000 licensed acupuncturist (more than any other state in the union) have years of intense study behind them. Each practitioner must graduate with four years of education at an approved school of Oriental medicine, including 1,548 hours of theory in both Western medicine and TCM. They must also complete 800 hours of clinical training and pass a California State exam. In New York, practitioners have to complete 4,050 hours (equivalent to three years) of education at an accredited university or college, with 60 semester hours focused in the sciences. They, too, must pass an exam.

In Indiana—one of the states in which acupuncture is not regulated—only medical doctors and doctors of osteopathy (O.D.) are allowed to perform acupuncture. Ironically, they are not required to take any training. In fact in most states, M.D.'s, D.O.'s, and chiropractors can practice acupuncture with little or no training at all. Meanwhile, those who set out to make TCM their life's work must endure years of rigorous training. This is a good argument for choosing only licensed acupuncturists to treat you. That way, you'll know you're getting someone who grasps the entire philosophy of TCM and how acupuncture fits into it.

The number grows every year, but currently there are 35 states that regulate acupuncture through state statutes. They are:

Alaska	Maine	Oregon
Arizona	Maryland	Pennsylvania
Arkansas	Massachusetts	Rhode Island
California	Minnesota	South Carolina
Colorado	Missouri	Texas
Connecticut	Montana	Utah
District of Columbia	Nevada	Vermont
Florida	New Hampshire	Virginia
Hawaii	New Jersey	Washington
Illinois	New Mexico	West Virginia
Iowa	New York	Wisconsin
Louisiana	North Carolina	

Both Kansas and Michigan allow the practice of acupuncture through a ruling from a medical board of examiners.

For information on the laws and regulations in your state, consult the National Acupuncture and Oriental Medicine Alliance at the Web address on page 95.

Certification and Accreditation

Several organizations contribute to the integrity of the profession by offering certification guidelines, a code of ethics, accreditation criteria, and national examinations or suggestions for state examinations. They include the following:

NCCAOM: National Certification Commission for Acupuncture and Oriental Medicine. Its mission is to "promote nationally recognized standards of competency and safety in acupuncture, Chinese herbology, and Oriental bodywork therapy, for the purpose of protecting the public." This organization offers the only educational, training, or examination criteria for licensure for certification in some states. Other states have their own criteria for education or examinations, but most practitioners seek NCCAOM certification. This certification earns the practitioner the title of diplomate in acupuncture (Dipl. Ac.), diplomate of Chinese herbology (Dipl. Ch. H.), or diplomate of Oriental bodywork therapy (Dipl. O.B.T.). The list of U.S. regulatory agencies affiliated with NCCAOM is lengthy—but all you need to know is that a practitioner who is certified through NCCAOM and holds the title of diplomate has met the highest standards in the field. For more information, call (703) 548-9004 or go to www.nccaom.org.

ACAOM: Accreditation Commission for Acupuncture and Oriental Medicine. Established in 1981, this is the group that decides whether a school is worthy of accreditation. The U.S. Department of Education recognizes ACAOM as the entity responsible for authorization. There are 46 schools in the United States and Canada that are either accredited or working on getting accreditation. There's more information on the Web at www.acaom.org.

AAOM: The American Association of Oriental Medicine. This association was formed in 1981 to "be the unifying force for American acupuncturists who are committed to high ethical and educational standards, and a well-regulated profession to ensure the safety of the public." They were instrumental in forming both NCCAOM and the National Council of Acupuncture Schools and Colleges. To find out more, call (888) 500-7999 or go to www.aaom.org.

AOMA: Acupuncture and Oriental Medicine Alliance. This organization keeps up with the state laws regarding acupuncture and provides a wide range of general information. Call (800) 345-1010 or go to www.acuall.org.

Finding the Right Practitioner

Everyone has different needs when looking for a health care practitioner. Some people care only about credentials. Others are more concerned about bedside manner. Everyone, no doubt, wants positive results. Finding the right fit with a TCM practitioner is no different, and it's important that you look for someone until you are certain you've found a good match.

> "Never go to a doctor whose office plants have died."
>
> —Erma Bombeck

The absolute best way to find a good practitioner is through word of mouth. I discovered Bing Lee through my friend Sara, who was historically leery of alternative medicine. Her infant had gone through a series of ear infections, and after many rounds of antibiotics, Sara's M.D. suggested an operation on her baby's eustachian tubes. The idea of putting her baby "under the knife" prompted Sara to seek alternative solutions.

She had heard success stories about Lee's work from other people in Aspen, Colorado, where she lives. With baby in tow, and in spite of her apprehensions, Sara visited Lee. After just a few minutes, Lee detected that the baby had an allergy to soymilk, as well as to the antibiotics he had been taking. The solution to the ear infections? No more soymilk, which would in turn mean no more antibiotics.

Upon making the dietary changes Lee suggested, Sara's baby immediately recovered from his ear infection, and as time went on, was no longer plagued by them. Consequently, Sara's worldview changed.

Knowing that I'm a believer in alternative medicine, she called me and recited her story with excitement. I was as thrilled as she was—and not just because her baby's ear infections were over (although that was great). Rather, if Sara believed in this guy, I knew there had to be something to him. I called him the next time something came up with my health, and I was as wowed as Sara was. Since I've had such great results with him, I've recommended him to as many people as I've heard complain about chronic troubles. Lee is a busy man.

That's word of mouth in action, and that's why it is more effective than 100 pricey television commercials. Nothing moves people faster than hearing real-life stories from friends about having found a trustworthy doctor, mechanic, hair stylist, or child care provider. That's because for most of us, health, independence, beauty, and our children are the most important parts of our lives (not necessarily in that order!). When we trust we're on to something good, we go for it. So, perk up your ears and start listening for good leads.

> "Three out of four doctors recommend another doctor."
>
> —Graffito

If you know someone who is already using a TCM practitioner, ask your friend for an honest assessment. What are the practitioner's strengths and weaknesses? Is your friend finding relief through the acupuncture, herbs, or other therapies? If so, that practitioner might be a good place to start. If not, keep looking (and read Chapters Seven through Nine).

If you don't know anyone who's getting acupuncture or working with a TCM professional, then look in the yellow pages or visit the local health food store. Most feature a bulletin board where people with alternative health practices can advertise their services. If none of these paths leads you in the right direction, there are a number of Internet sites that can help you locate qualified practitioners in your area. They include:

- ❦ American Association of Oriental Medicine: www.aaom.org
- ❦ Acupuncture and Oriental Medicine Alliance: www.acuall.org
- ❦ National Certification Commission for Acupuncture and Oriental Medicine: www.nccaom.org
- ❦ Council of Colleges of Acupuncture and Oriental Medicine: www.ccaom.org
- ❦ American Organization for Bodywork Therapies of Asia: www.healthy.net/aobta
- ❦ Acupuncture and Oriental Medicine Alliance: www.acupuncturealliance.org
- ❦ www.acupuncture.com
- ❦ www.healingpeople.com

Interviewing the Candidates

> "The most important part of acupuncture is the trusting relationship I have with [my practitioner], and the fact that it has made me much more aware of my body and its relationship to my spirit."
>
> —Chinese medicine survey participant
> as published in the *Journal of Alternative and Complementary Medicine* (Cassidy, 1998)

When you've located practitioners within your region, set up appointments to interview each of them and ask questions about their training, as well as their understanding of the principles of TCM. Utilizing acupuncture without understanding the complex world of Qi, yin and yang, Moisture, Blood, the organ network, the climates, and the elements is like trying to speak without the structure of sentences. Again, this may be why working with a licensed acupuncturist is the best choice. An M.D. or D.O. may know the basic language, but for acupuncture to be truly effective, the practitioner must grasp the relationship of the ailment to the rest of the physical, spiritual, and emotional bodies. Then again, if you live in a state that only allows M.D.'s and D.O.'s to perform acupuncture, it may still be worth moving forward as long as you have confidence in the doctor.

Now that you have a basic understanding of TCM, you can go to an interview with intelligent questions. Come up with a list of questions that specifically address your unique symptoms of IBS, as well. Ask how the practitioner thinks these symptoms may relate to other issues you are facing. Take no more than ten or fifteen minutes, but listen carefully and you will be able to tell if the individual has an overall understanding of TCM.

Other questions you may want to ask include:

- Where did you get your training? Did it include education in herbology as well as acupuncture?
- If you work with herbs, are they Chinese herbs, Western herbs, or a combination of both?

- How long did you study and/or apprentice?
- How long have you been in practice?
- Are you certified by NCCAOM?
- Do you have a state license? If not, do you have certification of any kind?
- Do you use disposable needles?
- What kind of acupuncture do you do? (Electro-acupuncture, moxibustion, and so on.)
- In addition to the traditional techniques for diagnosis, what other methods (such as muscle testing or hand modes) do you use to ascertain imbalance? (More on those methods later.)
- How long do the acupuncture sessions generally last?
- Do you accept insurance?

During your interview, notice how you feel in the individual's presence. Are you comfortable? Does he make you feel like your questions are welcome, or does he seem impatient? Does he listen as well as talk? Do you feel that he respects you? Do you feel comfortable venturing into new territory with him? Do you trust that you could open up to him about your emotional life? Ask what he charges and determine whether this will fit into your budget. Also, ask for references—especially from people who share a similar imbalance.

Choosing the path of TCM doesn't mean leaving the world of Western medicine behind. In fact, if you're like most of us who've made the leap, you will end up working with both. It's wise to find a TCM practitioner who isn't opposed to combining efforts with an M.D., or who will at least work to understand how to enhance what you're doing with Western medicine. You may find that Western medicine serves you quite nicely in certain acute areas of your health but that you want to approach chronic problems with TCM. Whatever choices you make, strive to work with professionals from both sides of the fence who appreciate your involvement and efforts to find solutions—regardless of whether the answers come from the East or the West.

To that end, be sure your practitioner of choice isn't stuck on one way of doing things. For example, if she has seen other patients with the same manifestations of IBS as yours, be sure she doesn't just leap into perfunctory treatment. Remember that your entire spectrum of influences and pattern of imbalance will be absolutely unique. The practitioner should rely on you, the individual, rather than familiar symptoms, to devise treatments. The beauty of TCM is that the practitioner is obligated to spend time with you to familiarize herself with your unique etiology. If she doesn't, you might consider moving on.

> "I consulted four different chiropractors until I found one that...was interested in my total health. No one was able to take the pain away from my neck until I started acupuncture. With the [antidepressant] I am taking now and the therapy with acupuncture, I am getting my life back together .... The regular M.D.'s did not take the pain away ... the chiropractic alone did not work, but together they worked very well."
>
> —Chinese medicine survey participant
> as published in the *Journal of Alternative
> and Complementary Medicine* (Cassidy, 1998)

Finally, ask how far in advance you need to schedule appointments. This can make the deciding difference in which practitioner you use. If you can only get into one person's office a month from now, you may opt for the person who can see you next week.

Upon discussing your needs, assessing the qualifications and character of the practitioners, and judging your comfort level with each one, you can then decide which individual suits you. That's when the journey really begins!

Personal Pay and Insurance Coverage

> "If you don't know where you're going, any road will do."
> —Chinese proverb

Slowly but surely, insurance companies are recognizing that patients who choose acupuncture are utilizing a cost-effective method of care—regardless of the condition for which they are being treated. Ultimately, cost-effective health care reaps more profits for insurance companies.

Even if your insurance company hasn't historically covered acupuncture and other TCM treatments, things may have changed by the time you pick up this book. Call your insurance agent to discover whether your company will indeed cover the costs. You can also ask your practitioner which insurance companies she works with. As of spring 2001, the following companies covered at least partial payment of acupuncture treatments:

- Aetna
- Blue Cross of California, Washington, and Alaska
- Blue Cross & Blue Shield of Oregon Aetna
- Cigna Health Care Plans in Washington State and Nebraska
- Disney World Services Metlife Network
- John Hancock Mutual Life
- Principal Mutual Life
- Prudential
- United Healthcare
- American Federation of Television and Radio Artists
- Director's Guild
- Motion Picture Industry Health Plan
- Screen Actor's Guild
- Writer's Guild
- Medical Savings Accounts (MSAs) as defined by the Internal Revenue Service (For self-employed people, an MSA can be underwritten by several different insurance companies. Even if the underwriter doesn't typically cover acupuncture, the IRS makes it legal for patients to do so with monies they've contributed to their account. If you have an MSA and aren't sure how to reimburse yourself for acupuncture treatments, contact your insurance agent.)

According to the National Acupuncture and Oriental Medicine Alliance, you may have more options for insurance coverage than you would initially think. Some policies pay for treatments only if they are recommended or performed by an M.D., but others will cover them if a licensed acupuncturist performs the procedure, when sessions are considered medically necessary, or for treatments of chronic pain. If your insurance company does cover the costs, be sure to read the fine print: There may be stipulations about the number of treatments they'll cover, who must perform them, and which conditions they'll cover. Probably the best bet is to work with your insurance agent and request a written policy regarding acupuncture.

If your carrier doesn't pay for treatments, take five minutes and write a letter to the state insurance commission. Send a copy to your state legislator and remind him or her that other states cover this valuable resource, and it's time your state does, too. As time goes on, more and more people will benefit from acupuncture treatments. When politicians and other elected officials hear about the need to include TCM in insurance policies, such coverage will likely become an option for everyone.

Until then, it's heartening to know that visits to an acupuncturist are usually not as expensive as those to medical doctors or specialists. Furthermore, you may find that after integrating acupuncture and other forms of TCM into your life, you'll save money by no longer needing as much care from medical doctors. This statement is backed up by the first in-depth, large-scale survey investigating why people use Chinese medicine and their satisfaction with it. Dr. Claire Cassidy reports in the *Journal of Alternative and Complementary Medicine* that "the majority [of survey participants] claimed that their use of non-Chinese care had decreased since they began receiving Chinese medicine care." The survey also reveals that of the 575 participants, acupuncture enabled:

- 84 percent to reduce their office visits to medical doctors
- 78.9 percent to reduce the use of prescription drugs
- 77.5 percent to see less of their physical therapist
- 77 percent to seek fewer reimbursements from their insurance company

- 70.1 percent to avoid surgery previously recommended by their M.D.'s (types of surgeries avoided included angioplasty, back, biopsy, cancer, carpal tunnel, colectomy, cyst removal, dental, ear-nose-throat, ear tubes, gallbladder, hand, hernia, hysterectomy, kidney stone, and knee)
- 58.5 percent to see less of their psychotherapist (Cassidy, 1998)

This all points to financial savings—especially since you don't have to pay for airfare to China to reap the benefits of using TCM.

Ben's Story, Age 53

I've had high cholesterol and a low thyroid for about ten years. I'm hypoglycemic, which turns me into a bear when I'm hungry. My wife says that I get angry easily anyway—whether I've had something to eat or not. Well, through the years I've spent thousands of dollars on tests for cholesterol and thyroid. Then I've had to pay for prescription drugs to keep those things in check. I've also been through a lot of therapy trying to get to the root of my anger. It's helped some, but it wasn't until I started working with TCM that I discovered that my cholesterol, thyroid, hypoglycemia, and anger were all related. My practitioner said acupuncture and herbs would do wonders for all those things. Well, sure enough, after about five sessions of acupuncture and taking some herbs, my last cholesterol and thyroid tests are normal. Plus, I no longer need those expensive prescription drugs. My wife says my bad temper has also softened. I'm eating a new diet that keeps me from getting shaky and upset when I'm hungry. I'm glad about all of it. But I'm really glad about the money I'm saving. My acupuncture treatments are half the price of visits to my M.D. I used to have to pay at least $100 per test for my cholesterol and thyroid, too. With all the money I'm saving, I figure I can take my wife out to more nice dinners.

"When I hear somebody sigh, 'Life is hard,' I am always tempted to ask, 'Compared to what?'"

—Sydney Harris

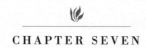

CHAPTER SEVEN

Beyond East and West: Taking a Deeper Look at Healing

We've covered a lot in this book. You know the Western definitions of irritable bowel syndrome (IBS), as well as the commonly prescribed "solutions." You know the fundamental philosophy and practice behind traditional Chinese medicine (TCM) and how it can help you. You know enough about acupuncture to lie on a table with needles sticking out of your belly and still maintain a smile. You even know how to track certain health imbalances by the map your tongue provides. Finally, you know how to go about finding a qualified TCM practitioner. So what's next? The next step, of course.

From this point forward, we're going to take you on a little journey by veering outside of the contemporary understanding of TCM. This will give you yet another chance to open your mind to some new and sometimes innovative concepts about illness, health, and treatment. These concepts are rooted in the ancient healing arts of China and India, but they have been diluted or nearly forgotten in the thousands of years that have passed since they were first developed. With this knowledge, you may choose to pursue a treatment that neither a Western doctor nor some TCM practitioners would suggest—only because they don't know about them.

"If the only tool you have is a hammer, you tend to see every problem as a nail."

—Abraham Maslow

Throughout this book we've been building a tool chest with which you can manage your IBS. What we're doing in this chapter is adding some new tools you won't find at any run-of-the-mill hardware store. A carpenter who possesses only a hammer and nails will not be as successful as one who has access to a variety of tools. Both may be able to build a house, but the one with the most tools will have an infinitely easier time building a safe, beautiful, and energy-efficient structure. The one with more tools will certainly be more prolific and will reap more rewards on a personal level. Likewise, the more tools you have, the greater your chances of eliminating the pain, inconvenience, and emotional distress of living with IBS.

Along the way, you may be introduced to concepts that seem a bit far-fetched. Try to stay open-minded. Just think how much fun you would have missed out on if you were still stuck with your initial reaction to how babies are made. At the time, it was incomprehensible and it sounded like something you'd never do. But life went on, and the rest is history. (Even though it's still incomprehensible!) The point is, regardless of your initial reactions to this stuff, attempt to suspend your doubts, consider what we're presenting, and then concern yourself with results. Because it's not how the methods work that really matters—it's that they *do* work. And isn't trying something new worth the possibility of living a healthy, symptom-free life?

Let's find out.

Symptoms versus Sources

As you know, Western medicine is good at looking at the parts (symptoms) of the imbalance. TCM is good at looking at the bigger picture (relationships) and is sensitive to the physical, mental, emotional, and spiritual bodies. So if ten people with the same IBS symptoms visited a medical doctor, they would likely be given the same diagnosis and the same treatment. If ten people with the same IBS symptoms visited a TCM practitioner, they would likely leave the office with ten different diagnoses and ten different treatments.

One practice looks at the pieces; the other looks at the whole. But there's another element involved in the dynamic of imbalance that few practitioners know how to spot. That's because it's an invisible part of the picture that symptoms don't reveal and conventional TCM diagnosis doesn't identify. The bottom line is that symptoms and diagnosis only signal that there is an imbalance—but they don't reveal the *actual source of* the imbalance. Chances are, these ten patients would walk out of both the M.D.'s and the TCM practitioner's offices without truly knowing what caused the imbalance.

"You can do acupuncture until you're blue in the face," says Bing Lee. "But if you don't get to the source of your imbalance, it won't do you any permanent good."

Think about it in this way: You're at home vacuuming while your son is in the bathroom blow-drying his hair, full blast. Your spouse is in the office at the back of the house with the air conditioner running full-tilt, and your daughter is in the garage pushing a power saw through some wood for her science project. Everything's fine until your mother throws a quickie meal into the microwave. Suddenly—POW!—and everything is silent. You've blown a fuse. So you go to the fuse box and throw back the circuit breaker. Energy's restored. Your son resumes his primping, your daughter goes about sawing, the air conditioner cranks up again, and you continue vacuuming. Everything is fine until your mother punches the button on the microwave. Then—POW!—no more energy, once again.

Having an imbalance is a lot like blowing a fuse. Getting an acupuncture treatment is a lot like throwing the circuit breaker so energy flows gracefully again. That is, until the source of your imbalance takes over again and your resources are either depleted or you're left seriously malfunctioning. So, you trundle back for another appointment. This leads to a long cycle of treatment and imbalance that is a familiar scenario for most people. Granted, these people are healthier than those who don't continue with or who have never had treatment. Even so, the treatments themselves don't identify the source and cannot keep you from blowing fuses; they can't heal you once and for all.

What can you do to find and maintain true health? Find a practitioner who can help you find the source!

The Surprise of Source

Milt is in his middle fifties. He has suffered with chronic diarrhea for thirty years and been to countless medical doctors who have tested him for everything under the sun. Nothing showed up, but the diarrhea didn't go away. He finally decided to try the alternative route and visited someone he had heard about that was helping people identify the sources of their problems.

The man Milt visited was a TCM practitioner, but he didn't take Milt's pulse or look at his tongue. Rather, he asked Milt a series of questions about his diet, his home environment, and his personal hygiene products. As the practitioner asked the questions, one of his hands was in constant movement, making gestures that resemble the sign language used by the deaf. The questions continued, especially those regarding personal hygiene products, until he asked:

"What kind of deodorant do you use?"

Puzzled, Milt told him.

"How long have you been using it?"

"I don't know. For as long as I can remember. Thirty years."

The practitioner nodded his head and smiled. He told Milt to stop using the deodorant because Milt was allergic to it. Milt figured the practitioner was nuts. Then Milt received an acupuncture treatment.

Milt decided to give up the deodorant because he had nothing to lose and was desperate for relief from his pain. He visited the practitioner two weeks later and reported that his diarrhea was virtually gone. For the first time in thirty years, he was experiencing regular bowels. Milt threw away that deodorant.

❦❦❦

When she was five years old, Tammy began complaining of headaches. By the time she was six and still complaining of them, her mother became worried. After nightmarish worst-case scenarios kept floating through her mind, Tammy's mother finally called a doctor. The doctor suggested that Tammy be put through routine tests so they could rule out the obvious horror stories. But between the high deductible for the family's health insurance and the idea of subjecting her daughter to a battery of tests that might scare her, Tammy's mother opted to start with an alternative approach. She found a practitioner who diagnosed using muscle testing, which is a form of energy work.

Tammy sat in a chair with one arm raised to shoulder level while the practitioner touched certain points on her body. The doctor asked Tammy to resist as he pushed down on her arm and asked some questions. After a few moments, the practitioner deduced that the headaches were due to something in Tammy's diet. He asked several more questions specific to the girl's diet, and shortly thereafter he concluded that Tammy was having an allergic reaction to both cow's milk and fruit juice. He suggested that Tammy only drink soymilk and stay clear of fruit juice for a few months.

Since eliminating those things from her diet, Tammy hasn't had any headaches.

❦❦❦

Martha is an active, 42-year-old woman. She runs her own business, has small children, and participates in her community. She eats well and exercises regularly. She enjoys wine with dinner and occasionally drinks bourbon. But Martha had trouble sleeping and was often awakened by hot flashes. Once she was awake, she had trouble getting back to sleep because "turbo-brain" would kick in and she couldn't keep her thoughts quiet. Ironically, during the day, her body temperature was typically cold and she couldn't seem to warm up. On most days, Martha experienced sharp, constant headaches that started by about 4 p.m and lasted until she went to bed. She wondered if the headaches were due to her thyroid. She had been on thyroid medication for seven years, but her last tests had come up normal, and her doctor had taken her off the medication. She was able to function with these symptoms, but because of the lack of sleep and nagging headaches, she decided to seek help.

Martha had been to an energy healer before with good results. She returned to him with her inventory of ailments and waited for the practitioner to fire off his questions.

Martha was convinced that she had an allergic reaction to the wine, but after examining her, the practitioner said that wasn't a problem. Rather, he said, she was low on pituitary. Martha questioned that, stating that her thyroid had traditionally been the problem, but that her tests were normal. The practitioner explained that the pituitary is the master of the thyroid, and if it isn't in balance, symptoms of thyroid deficiencies will emerge, but the root of the problem is not with the thyroid. He said that pituitary imbalances also cause hormonal imbalances, and those were the reason for the hot flashes. What's more, pituitary symptoms are typically linked with worry and overthinking, which can cause sleeplessness. No argument there. Martha left with a supplement of pituitary gland.

One month later, Martha returned to the practitioner and said all of her symptoms had ceased, except for the headaches. Upon asking more questions and checking her energy patterns, the practitioner said she should avoid the bourbon, but that there was something more.

"What kind of coffee do you drink?"

Before she could answer, he told her the exact brand.

"How did you know?" she asked.

According to that practitioner, a lot of people have reactions to certain strong brands of coffee. He told her to change brands. She did— and stopped the bourbon—after which the headaches disappeared.

❧❧❧

Elizabeth visited an energy healer complaining of pains in her lower back. They weren't so serious that she couldn't function, but they weren't something that she wanted to live with. Through his techniques, the practitioner concluded that she had a reaction to something electrical. No, she didn't use a blow dryer for her hair. No electric shavers. Her bedside clock was battery-operated. No electric blankets. But yes, she did sleep on a waterbed and it did have an electric heater attached to it.

"It's broken. Get another one," the practitioner said.

She did, and the back pains went away.

❦❦❦

There are hundreds of stories like this. They're intriguing because they go against all logic and scientific reasoning—but they all have happy endings! Each one of these people was able to eliminate symptoms by identifying the source of their problem and implementing a treatment that dealt with the source rather than the symptoms. When the source is identified, true and lasting healing can occur.

Harnessing Energy Healing

In a June 1997 report of the Council on Scientific Affairs from the American Medical Association on alternative medicine, energy healing is described by its proponents as "one of the oldest forms of healing known to humankind." Theories related to this practice involve transfer of energy from healer to patient in unknown ways, either from a supernatural entity or by manipulating the body's own "energy fields." Over 25 terms are used in various cultures to describe this life force. Energy healers incorporate a holistic focus into therapy. They promote their methods as useful for handling stress and for the general improvement of appetite, indigestion, and various emotional states, plus the treatment of conditions such as eating disorders, irritable bowel syndrome, and premenstrual syndrome.

Energy, Frequencies, and Diagnostic Dialoguing

TCM comes closer to identifying the source of imbalances than does Western medicine, but that is still not the objective. Rather, the objective of TCM is to balance or unblock the flow of Qi. This goes a long way toward helping people recover, but still, there are people for whom it doesn't work. Likewise, Chinese and Western herbs don't work for everyone. Drugs don't work for everyone, either. This begs the question "Why isn't there such thing as a magic bullet? Especially when all symptoms are the same?"

As the stories we've related illustrate, the source of imbalance can spring from a multitude of different arenas. Let's return, for a moment, to those ten people who all share the same symptoms of IBS. According to Lee, drugs may work for two of the individuals, if the source of their problem is bacterial. Two others may have success with herbs or enzymes, if the root of their imbalance is poor digestion. Drinking ten to twelve glasses of water daily could alleviate the problem for another two people whose systems are dehydrated from excess caffeine intake. The next two would find relief in meditation and flower essence remedies because the source of their IBS is emotional stress and repressed anger. Finally, the last two may have a thyroid or adrenal deficiency for which natural or herbal supplementation provides the cure. But if all of these individuals— with the exact same symptoms—were put on any single treatment, then only 20 percent would find relief. If people experience lasting relief without identifying the source, they are either fitting into a statistical average or they're just plain lucky.

"In TCM, you could diagnose irritable bowel syndrome as Gallbladder Qi stagnation, Large Intestine Qi stagnation, Stomach Qi deficiency, or a host of other names, depending on the exact manifestations," Lee explains. "In Western medicine, they usually just call it IBS, or maybe an infection or overactive bacteria. But no matter what you call it, whether it's a TCM term or what medical doctors name it, it comes down to energy."

In fact, everything is energy. Science doesn't argue with that. Lee elaborates on the idea by stressing that everything has a unique energy pattern, vibration, or frequency. This means that diarrhea is an energy; constipation is an energy; bloating, gas, pain, and all the things we call symptoms or imbalances can each be identified as a specific energy. Following this train of thought, every hormone has an energy, every organ, every limb on our bodies, every thought in our heads. So do the foods we eat, the cleansing products we use, the chairs we sit in, the cars we drive, the air we breathe, the people we hang out with. No matter what we call a thing, when you reduce it to its purest essence, it is a form of energy. Everything is energy. Everything.

Through language we *label* these different energies—from the most dense energies, as found in the physical, tangible world, to the most refined energies, which are unmanifested. We call something a rock, but it is in essence dense energy. Something less dense is called a tree. We give our feelings and emotions labels, but they are in truth just refined energy. And we give the most refined energy of all the name of God, Allah, Jesus, Buddha, or whichever name has been given to that energy that attracts you.

In the stories told here, each practitioner was either in communication with the energy of the patient's body and imbalance or was actually experiencing it. Knowing how to do this enables the healer to pick up on specific vibrational frequencies that the imbalance is sending out as an SOS. And from that, the balancing energy can also be identified. In ancient times—and in rare cases these days—the healer does nothing more than hold a hand over the patient's head, name the imbalance, trace the source, and offer the appropriate solution. Even though this may sound like part science-fiction, part fairytale, these abilities have been around forever, and as long as there are receptive people, they will continue to be.

Dialoguing with energy is the lost healing art we referred to earlier in the chapter. Although the concepts aren't often part of casual conversations at hospital fundraisers, those unique individuals who choose to go beyond what they learned in medical or TCM school continue to keep the art alive. These people are explorers, and they emerge from all circles of thought. In essence, they come to realize that something is missing from what they are doing, that there is more. So, they go deeper with their studies into the nature of and relationship between health and imbalance. In essence, they take the next step, and the next, and the next, as they devote themselves to becoming true healers. By sharing this information with you, we're giving you the opportunity to go deeper with your healing process.

It worked for Nathan, a healthy man in his mid-thirties. He eats well, doesn't smoke or drink, exercises regularly, and is pleased with his work and home life. In mid-January, he began to experience excruciating abdominal pain. After missing a few days of work, he finally went to his doctor. They did an upper GI, lower GI, the whole gamut of tests. But according to his tests, Nathan was as healthy as he'd always been. The pain continued, but Nathan decided painkillers weren't the answer. After three consecutive weeks of debilitating pain, Nathan visited Lee.

Lee asked a series of questions about Nathan's lifestyle, eating habits, environment, emotional life, and personal hygiene products. As Nathan answered the questions, Lee engaged in a dialogue with Nathan's body by using mudras, or hand modes. (This is the "sign language" mentioned earlier.) As he listened to Nathan's answers, Lee continued the hand modes until he was able to receive a signal from Nathan's body. When he identified the source, Lee experienced a physical response. After several minutes of hand modes, Lee asked Nathan if he used cologne. Nathan replied, "I don't usually, but I got some for Christmas and I've been using it ever since."

The pains started in January, several weeks after Christmas. Bingo. Lee's body *experienced* that this was the source of the problem.

There was no need for treatment. There was only the need to eliminate the cologne. Two weeks later—after closing the top on the cologne very tightly—the pain vanished, and Nathan is back to his healthy self.

Dialoguing with energy is probably both a gift and a learned skill. To develop his abilities, in addition to completing studies and becoming a licensed diplomate, Lee studied with several different teachers, including a chiropractor, who know how to speak the language. Lee also attributes his insights to thirty years of meditation.

Much of what you'll read in the following pages is Lee's interpretation of and experience with this nearly lost healing art. Other healers may explain or do things in slightly different manners. That's fine, because each practitioner operates from his or her own knowledge base.

Testing the Limits, or the Limits of Tests

If you're one of those people that holds fast to clinical trials, test results, and conclusive scientific data, you probably think what we're saying is a bunch of hogwash. Truthfully, we have no quarrel with tests and scientific studies because they serve a very valuable purpose. Even so, there is a limit to that purpose, which is what most people don't realize. Those limits are not something steadfast scientists talk about, but we're going to. (I bet you already knew that.)

Let's start by agreeing with the rest of the world that our bodies are made up of bones, blood, muscles, organs, tissue, and so on. Our bodies function because of chemistry. There's also emotional chemistry. Surely, if you've ever fallen in love (and it was mutual), you felt both the emotional and physical chemistry. Chemistry is energy at play.

Chemistry is usually talked about in physical terms. It's what we can grasp, see, touch, test, validate through science, and so on. Much of America's health care system is based on what has been learned through scientific probing into physical chemistry.

Then there are snowflakes. Yes, snowflakes. Everyone knows there are no two snowflakes alike. That's as incomprehensible as anything else you could imagine because there are billions and billions of snowflakes. Even though snowflakes contain the same ingredients, we know that not a single one shares the same pattern.

Guess what, folks—this holds true for people, too. Look at your fingerprints and marvel at the fact that they are uniquely yours. Yes, we have the same ingredients. No, we don't have the same patterns of imbalance, as we've discussed. We also don't necessarily have the same patterns of balance. Chew on this over your next fiber shake:

Your baseline of health may be different than other people's, meaning that your body chemistry could have different requirements than the average Joe (or Jane). You may need more thyroid, for example, even if blood tests indicate that your thyroid is within a healthy range. Tests provide ranges based on a statistical average. So, according to the tests, you could fall into what's considered normal, but still need more thyroid to function at 100 percent.

Chance as a Scientific Fact

". . . It is imperative to cast off certain prejudices of the Western mind. It is a curious fact that such a gifted and intelligent people as the Chinese has never developed what we call science. Our science, however, is based upon the principle of causality, and causality is considered to be an axiomatic truth. But a great change in our standpoint is setting in. What Kant's *Critique of Pure Reason* failed to do is being accomplished by modern physics. The axioms of causality are being shaken to their foundations: we know now that what we term natural laws are merely statistical truths and thus must necessarily allow for exceptions. We have not sufficiently taken into account as yet that we need the laboratory with its incisive restrictions in order to demonstrate the invariable validity of natural law. If we leave things to nature, we see a very different picture: every process is partially or totally interfered with by chance, so much so that under natural circumstances a course of events absolutely conforming to specific laws is almost an exception."

—Excerpt from Carl Jung's
introduction to *The I Ching*,
or *Book of Changes*

Tests are valuable because they represent an average of many people and they provide a form of measurement. They can be applicable to a great many people, but we must be mindful of the limitations of what they measure, or more to the point, what they don't measure. They don't show the relationship between the ingredients that add up to good health. They don't consider the millions of people who don't fit within the standard. In this way, medical tests are very similar to standardized tests in schools. These tests cannot reveal the innate intelligence of a creative, artistic, musical, or scientifically gifted child. They cannot measure the intelligence of children who learn intuitively, kinesthetically, or through auditory means. A very smart child often gets answers wrong because the logic of the tests doesn't fit within his or her curious and more inquisitive mind. This is why tests of all kinds fall short.

"There are so many people with thyroid problems," Lee says. "I tell them that's what they need and they say, 'My tests are fine. My doctor says I don't need thyroid.' I say, 'Those tests don't apply to your system.' They take a thyroid supplement for a month, come back, and report that they feel like a million bucks."

Not everyone fits the numbers. Lee explains that a qualitative approach rather than a quantitative approach to finding and maintaining balance recognizes the individual, not a statistical average.

Even for strictly physical conditions, tests are not always as absolute as we may want to believe. Lee tells the story of a patient who had a torn rotator cuff. She went to one set of reputable experts who did an MRI and employed a series of different technological means to study the problem from a scientific point of view. Their conclusion was that the patient needed surgery. But before that, she wanted another opinion. (Speaking of which, why would we ever get a second opinion if the conclusions that could be drawn from medical science were absolute?) So, she went to a different reputable bunch of experts. They also performed an MRI, along with a series of scientifically based diagnostic tests. Their conclusion—based on the same or similar scientific data as the first set of experts—was that the patient did not need surgery. What's absolute and scientific about that? Nothing. It came down to interpretation, and science is a product of interpretation based on statistical average.

Chronic problems are usually an indication that you don't fit the numbers. Chances are, you've been treated based on statistics rather than your individual baseline. And keep in mind that this baseline includes not just your body but also your mind and spirit.

Tests don't divulge the emotional components that contribute to illness. You already know from the first half of this book that emotional energies can greatly impact physical conditions. Your personal and unique baseline is affected by all the energies at play in your life. No test can measure these influences, nor can they address the healing or transforming power of love. But most people know, in their heart of hearts, that love is the greatest sustaining energy around.

Brenda's Story, Age 44

Back when I was just thirty years old, I began to experience non-stop diarrhea. It was so bad that I needed to wear a diaper at night. I was a registered nurse working in a 900-bed hospital in Washington, DC. The stress of the job was horrible. I worked with a lot of AIDS patients, then I'd come home to the demands of three young children. I took all the usual medical tests, and everything came up normal. That's when I realized my body was probably reacting to stress.

I took some time off. I visited more doctors. I kept getting the same message from them, but after several months off of work, the symptoms stopped. I quit my old job and started at a smaller hospital that had a better pace and fewer high-maintenance patients. I only worked part-time so I could be with the kids. My health returned.

Then, three years later, my husband committed suicide. I had four kids and no choice but to go back to work as a nurse, full-time. It wasn't long before the diarrhea started up again. A dentist told me he thought it might be related to the mercury in my fillings, so I had them removed and started a program to cleanse my body from the effects of the mercury. But I had a toxic reaction to whatever I was taking, and then everything got worse—bloating, distension, gas, and more diarrhea. I was in horrible shape. I looked about six months pregnant, couldn't work because of the diarrhea, and eventually could barely walk. One doctor accused me of secretly using laxatives so I could get all the attention I was demanding. Meanwhile, I was expelling two to three liters of diarrhea per day and falling into a horrible depression. Finally, another doctor told me that I was disabled and had better learn to live with it.

That was when I decided to look into alternative medicine. There was no way I was going to leave my kids with a bedridden mother. There was also no way I was going to go back into nursing once I was well. I started with acupuncture, and that helped a lot. But I found that what worked for me was a combination of chiropractic work, acupuncture, and a less-stressful job.

After years of chasing down help from the field in which I worked, I finally found relief in TCM and chiropractic. I know the cause of all this is stress, so I keep a very close watch on myself. I've started a new business selling herbal products to people and have ended up making more money than my very best years as a nurse. My kids have their Mom back, and I have my life back.

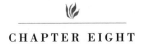

CHAPTER EIGHT

Self-Evaluation: Taking a Journey to the Unexpected

The first and most important step toward working with your irritable bowel syndrome (IBS) from an energetic point of view is to start over. Look at your condition with new eyes, and think about it with a mind for complete and final healing. Commit to exploring new ways of working with it—no matter how foreign they may seem. In short, relinquish the diagnoses you've received, as well as what you've been told to do. That may sound radical, but if what you've been told has limited your options for treatment and if what you've tried hasn't worked yet, it probably never will. Now's the time to try an entirely new approach with the intent of finding the key that unlocks the deadbolt IBS has on your health.

This is an individual process because each person is like a walking chemistry set; each one of us has strengths and weaknesses all our own. As we've discussed, your IBS symptoms may be precisely the same as your friend's, but hers may be caused by a combination of dehydration and low thyroid. Yours may be due to an allergy to mouthwash. Unfolding the mystery of why you're experiencing the problem requires that you stop focusing on symptoms or diagnosis.

Instead, look at yourself as an individual with a totally unique makeup and etiology. You are an individual who is affected by as many variables as there are influences in your life; you are someone who may not fit a prescribed model that says you should be healthy. No more referring back to statistics, to what worked for IBS study participant #14, to wishing the drugs you tried had continued to give you relief. From this point forward, we're going to help you look at *yourself.* You as a whole and separate entity. Treating *you*—rather than your symptoms—is the objective, and finding the source of your imbalance is the goal.

Noticing the Bigger Picture

We're on a mission to evaluate what's here, now, and uniquely yours. Although it may seem overwhelming at times, this mission is not impossible. Begin by walking through each day with an alert eye for what upsets your system. Take an inventory of all the influences in your life, beginning with what you are closest to and then extending into your larger environment. Keep an IBS journal in which you can record observations and thoughts. As you go through your day, pay attention to the foods you eat and to how your condition changes in the various environments in which you spend your time. Are your symptoms worse at work, at home, at your parent's house, or at your sweetheart's place? What emotions do you tend to experience at each place? Do symptoms act up more in the morning, afternoon, or night? Does sitting in one particular chair rather than another relieve some of the pain? Does cloudy weather make things better or worse? Does eating lettuce set it off?

Before now, you may not have thought about the many variables that could be contributing to your condition, so you might have missed some clues. Becoming aware of the range of possibilities of what could be aggravating your situation can awaken you to specific sources that you've dismissed before. Remain alert, tune in to your body, and notice as many environmental and emotional factors as you can when you're under abdominal siege.

If you feel that you've already analyzed your situation to death and simply don't want to survey it anymore, that's fine. Whether you choose to begin an inventory on your own or not, you should ultimately work with a professional who has learned the art of energy dialogue. He or she can act as the guide as you explore the universe in which you live while pursuing the elusive gold at the end of the rainbow—the source of your IBS.

Finding and Working with an Energy Healer

You may already know an energy healer, without even realizing it! People who dialogue with energy don't walk around with feathers and bones in their hair, don't have magic wands, and don't live in caves tucked between the pine trees. Many of them do work in alternative health care professions such as TCM, chiropractic, massage therapy, or as naturopathic and homeopathic doctors. Although not everyone in these fields knows the language we're discussing, probably all of them have heard of muscle testing and Kinesiology, the most common names for dialoguing with energy.

Kinesiology isn't what the ancient Chinese and Indians used, but it's what most practitioners today rely on, it has been proven effective, and it is used around the world. According to Kinesiologists United, an association for professionals who employ muscle testing, the original method was developed in 1964 by Dr. George Goodheart. This "goodhearted" doctor "discovered that manual muscle testing could be used to obtain diagnostic information directly from the body of a patient. He called this new way of communicating with the body Applied Kinesiology, and it started a revolution in health care that is still gaining momentum."

Indeed, since 1964, a number of different schools have sprouted out of Applied Kinesiology, each with a slightly different approach to communicating with the body. When searching for a practitioner, you may hear of any number of techniques, including Applied Physiology, BioSet, Clinical Kinesiology, Health Kinesiology, Integrative Kinesiology, Touch for Health, Jaffee-Mellor Technique,

Kinergetic, Wellness Kinesiology, and more. To keep things simple, when you're shopping for your new practitioner, simply ask if she or he uses muscle testing. That says it all, regardless of the technique.

There are no educational requirements for using muscle testing as a guide for diagnosis, so you're going to have to use different criteria to determine whether the practitioner you've found is a good one. Like anything else, there are good ones and bad ones and lots of in-between ones. As we suggested before, start by asking friends if they know of and have gone to a practitioner who uses muscle testing. It's becoming more and more common in alternative medicine circles, and you may find out that your next-door neighbor has been using one for years.

A visit to a practitioner who uses muscle testing will be unlike any other office visit you've been on. To begin with, while you're either sitting or lying down, the practitioner will ask you to raise your arm (to the side or straight up, depending on your position). Then, she'll apply pressure to your arm while asking you to resist her push. All she's doing at this point is testing the strength of the muscle. While you continue to resist her push, she will internally ask your body a series of questions. (Remember: Thoughts are energy, and all she has to do is *think* the question for it to be communicated to your body.) For each answer, she will push down on your arm. She may also use her other hand to touch trigger points on your body as she asks the questions and pushes on your arm.

Unless she asks the questions aloud, you will have no idea what the practitioner is asking, but at a certain point, you may suddenly be unable to resist the pressure she is exerting on your arm. This is a significant signal that your body is sending to her.

When a practitioner is dialoguing with your body, she phrases her questions so that your body can give a yes or no answer. For example, she may start by asking, "Is the diarrhea due to an excess within the system?"

If you are able to hold your arm up, the answer is no. At that point, she will move on and ask another question, such as "Is the diarrhea due to a deficiency?" Again, if you can hold your arm up, the answer is still no. But if you cannot resist her push and your arm loses its strength, the answer is yes. In that case, she will then start a series of questions about which deficiency your body is experiencing, and you will again be able to resist her push until she asks a question that is answered "yes."

The answers your body provides can go beyond diagnosis to reveal the cause or source of your imbalance. This is the dialogue that can break the cycle of your illness. This is the vital step that is missed in both Western medicine and some forms of TCM.

When you first expose yourself to muscle testing, you might be tempted to laugh it off. You might even try to maintain a strong arm when your arm is actually weak and trying to relay an important message. Your mind may play all kinds of tricks on you. That's normal, given that this approach is quite a departure from the medical culture we're all accustomed to. But if your intent is to get better, you will ignore the skepticism, trust the process, and listen to the answers the practitioner has received. The only way to know if muscle testing works is to allow the process to occur with as much honesty as possible and then act on the information the practitioner receives from your body.

Now, let's get into what you can use as the blueprint for pinpointing imbalance.

Discerning the Source and Providing Solutions

Not all of the ancient wisdom from the healing arts has been lost over the years. Most alternative practitioners know that when physical imbalances show up, the source can be due to something physical in nature, something emotional, or a combination of emotional and physical upsets. Regardless of the source or sources, four different types of agitation can result: superficial, infection, deficiency, or excess.

The way to restore balance to your system is to follow the principle that yin and yang reveal: For every energy, there is a counter-energy. If there's a deficiency in the system, add what's missing to the body. If there's something toxic in the system, eliminate it from the body. When you work with a practitioner who knows how to dialogue with energy, your body will reveal what's out of balance, and the practitioner can treat it with elimination or an energetic opposite. The solutions are often very simple.

Deficiencies and excesses cause about 99 percent of all imbalances. Below, you'll find an overview of potential irritants, as well as solutions that reestablish balance. Take this information with you when visiting your practitioner. Ask him or her to muscle test you while going through this list to help determine the root cause of your IBS, as well as the best ways to treat it.

SUPERFICIAL IMBALANCES

Superficial imbalances and those based in infection are typically caused by an overload of stress. These problems show up in a variety of ways—including bouts of IBS—but they can be alleviated with simple strategies. Go to the beach for a day. Give up cleaning the house for a week. Pop open some wine and order takeout for dinner. Quit answering the phone for a weekend and put your nose in a good novel. Muscle testing won't necessarily reveal these specific answers, but it will indicate that you need rest. Superficial imbalances simply mean you're not giving yourself enough downtime. Sometimes people figure out that they need a break before the stress overwhelms them and erupts into something worse. If you're feeling anxious, overwhelmed, emotional, angry, or simply exhausted, try some downtime. If you're paying attention, you won't need to visit a practitioner when you get signals that there's a need to stop. Simply stop, which, of course, is the ideal response.

Since we live in such a demanding world, it's wise to be ever mindful of your emotional and physical states. Instead of "powering through" the signals that you need a break, go ahead and take a break. Respect yourself and your body enough to know that yin energy—or quiet time, relaxation, and doing nothing—is as important as eating and breathing. You cannot live in a fast-paced yang state all the time, or you will worsen chronic problems and develop acute ones. We'll address emotional issues later, but for now—and always—pay attention to what your body and spirit need. Allow for balance in how you live your life. You don't have to fork out a single cent to a practitioner to learn that the best medicine you can take is a day off.

INFECTION-BASED IMBALANCES

You know this type of imbalance. Sneezing, coughing, fever, ear-aches. It's *the crud*, and it's because of an infection. There are two types of infection: bacterial and viral.

Antibiotics work for bacterial infections, but not viral ones. Be careful not to become dependent on antibiotics. Surely, you've read the cautionary tales about how bacteria are becoming immune to the fighting forces within antibiotics. That's simply due to overuse. Also, beware if you experience chronic infections. This means something else is going on, and it may be appropriate to work with an energy healer to help figure out what's causing them. They could be triggered by an allergic reaction to foods (as was the case for Sara's baby) or by a toxin in your environment. It's especially important to find the source if your child has recurrent infections. Kids who take too many antibiotics become adults with seriously compromised immune systems. Remember, too, that you may be creating or exacerbating another imbalance by taking pharmaceutical drugs too often.

There's not a lot you can do for viral infections except let them run their course. Drink lots of water and rest as much as possible. Also, keep a good supply of Chinese herbs that boost the immune system. (Ask at your local health food store for recommendations to treat specific symptoms.) They will help ward off both bacterial and viral infections and fight any infection your body is currently battling.

DEFICIENCIES

When your body is missing an essential ingredient, your overall chemistry is thrown off, and this can cause troubles of all kinds. Deficiencies are usually hormonal, biological, or dietary in nature.

Hormonal deficiencies include those of the pituitary, thyroid, and adrenal glands.

You may not think hormones have anything to do with what goes on inside your gut, but remember: Everything that goes on within your system will affect your system's overall chemistry. It's just as likely that you have IBS due to a hormonal imbalance as anything else.

Pituitary, thyroid, and adrenal deficiencies can display very similar symptoms and share certain others, such as chronic fatigue. Still, if your imbalance is hormonally based, it's important to single out which hormone is behind your condition so you can treat it accordingly. Each one of these deficiencies can be balanced with nonprescription, bovine supplements available through your health care practitioner. Although your practitioner should muscle test you to determine whether you have a hormonal deficiency, here are some common (although not absolute) indications of which hormones may be lacking.

Emotional and Lifestyle Indicators
of Hormonal Imbalance

IF YOU ARE:	THEN YOU MAY NEED MORE:
• A worrier	
• An analyzer	
• Full of mind chatter	
• Having trouble letting things go	Pituitary
• Unable to focus	
• Excessively tired	
• Having irregular menstrual periods or unexplainable hot flashes	
• Experiencing unusual memory loss	
• Unable to sleep because unable to stop thinking about things	

(continued)

Emotional and Lifestyle Indicators
of Hormonal Imbalance

IF YOU ARE:	THEN YOU MAY NEED MORE:
• A workaholic • Always on the go • Experiencing tightness in your chest or palpitations • Aware of numbness in your hands and arms • Prone to allergies • Excessively tired • Trying to do it all	Thyroid
• Fearful • Living with chronic lower back pain • Urinating more than you think you should • Excessively tired	Adrenal

Biological and dietary deficiencies can also affect your system's balance. These deficiencies may include:

❧ Amino acids
❧ Beneficial fat
❧ Beneficial yeast
❧ Enzymes

- Essential fatty acids
- Friendly bacteria
- Hydrochloric acid production
- Vitamins and minerals
- Water

If your imbalance isn't related to hormones, working with an energy healer will provide answers to a host of dietary considerations. If an energy healer finds you have a deficiency in one or several of these categories, try supplementing with what Lee has found works to establish balance (see the chart below). You should be able to find these items at any health food store. Ask the practitioner to test your body to see which supplement it needs.

IF YOU ARE LOW ON:
Hydrochloric acid (HCL)

THE REASON MAY BE:
You may have an underproduction of HCL. This leads to acid indigestion, acid reflux, and a hot and sour feeling in your stomach. The food inside your stomach is turning rancid because you don't have enough acid to break it down.

TRY SUPPLEMENTING WITH:
Betaine HCL (a supplemental form of hydrochloric acid)

IF YOU ARE LOW ON:
Friendly bacteria

THE REASON MAY BE:
When you take antibiotics, you kill the beneficial bacteria along with the bad. The good bacteria in your gut are necessary for proper digestion. That's why you should always take acidophilus when on antibiotics, but talk to your health care provider about how and when to take it.

TRY SUPPLEMENTING WITH:
Acidophilus

(continued)

IF YOU ARE LOW ON:
Beneficial yeast

THE REASON MAY BE:
Antibiotics. *Candida albicans* is a fancy word for the yeast that lives in mouths, vaginas, and intestinal tracts. Just like bacteria, yeast is a natural and essential ingredient for efficient digestion. Too many antibiotics can upset the balance of yeast in your system.

TRY SUPPLEMENTING WITH:
Brewer's yeast

IF YOU ARE LOW ON:
Essential fatty acids

THE REASON MAY BE:
Too little healthy fat in your diet. We talked a lot about the importance of EFAs in Chapter One, and we'll be talking more about them in the next chapter. You might be surprised to learn how important they are, and that too little fat could be the root of your problem.

TRY SUPPLEMENTING WITH:
The omega-3 and -6 fatty acids, including canola, corn, fish, flaxseed, grapeseed, safflower, soybean, sunflower seed, walnut, and wheat germ oils. Also, the gamma-linolenic acids including black currant, borage, and evening primrose oils. You can also get a boost of these valuable oils by eating fresh-water fish including mackerel, salmon, sardines, and tuna about three times a week. Chicken, eggs, and turkey also contain EFAs.

IF YOU ARE LOW ON:
Amino acids

THE REASON MAY BE:
You're eating too few amino-acid-containing foods. Amino acids make up the proteins that create enzymes, hormones, and neurotransmitters. We get 22 amino acids from foods, but when they hit the chemistry within our bodies, they are transformed into 50,000 different molecules that enable us to function.

TRY SUPPLEMENTING WITH:
Glutamine, an amino acid that is especially helpful with digestion.

(continued)

IF YOU ARE LOW ON:
Enzymes

THE REASON MAY BE:
Not enough raw vegetables. Among other duties, enzymes are the little guys (made of protein) responsible for breaking down food so it can move swiftly through your digestive tract. It makes sense that if you have a problem with digestion, you may have an enzyme deficiency. By the way, canned foods are stripped of enzymes so they will have a longer shelf life. If you're highly dependent on canned or premade foods, you aren't getting enough enzymes.

TRY SUPPLEMENTING WITH:
A multienzyme product that includes ingredients such as carbohydrase, amylase, protease, lipase, cellulase, bromelain, super oxidate dimutase, and catalase.

IF YOU ARE LOW ON:
Vitamins and minerals

THE REASON MAY BE:
Poor diet or quality of food intake. You probably know how significant vitamins and minerals are to your health. The bottom line is, you can't live without them. Ask your practitioner to test your body to find out specifically which vitamins and minerals it craves.

TRY SUPPLEMENTING WITH:
Multivitamin and mineral supplement. Look into B vitamins in particular to aid with digestion.

IF YOU ARE LOW ON:
Water

THE REASON MAY BE:
You don't drink enough! Filtered water is best, but faucet water is better than nothing!

TRY SUPPLEMENTING WITH:
Ten to 12 glasses per day. If you're not used to drinking this much and find the need to urinate inconvenient, rest assured that your body will get used to processing that much water and you'll have to go less often after a while. Water is nothing to ignore. It's essential to a healthy body.

EXCESSES

We all know that too much of something—even a good thing—can lead to uncomfortable consequences. What we rarely hear about and what we pay little attention to, however, is that everyone's system is sensitive to *something*—even in the smallest doses. Remember Nathan? He was the picture of health until he applied the Christmas cologne to his skin. Although he only dabbed it on in tiny amounts, his system was super-sensitive to it. Just a tablespoon was toxic enough to tie his colon into knots. You don't need excessive amounts of a substance for it to be toxic to your system; the fact that it is toxic to you means that any amount is excessive.

Pinpointing excesses of toxins can be somewhat more time-consuming than identifying deficiencies. There are so many influences in the environment to which you could have an allergy or sensitivity. Here's a breakdown of common environmental elements that can be the source of a toxic reaction.

INTERNAL ENVIRONMENT

- Bacteria
- Fungus
- Parasites
- Yeast

EXTERNAL ENVIRONMENT: DIRECT CONTACT

- After-shave lotion
- Air freshener
- Alcohol
- Animals
- Any kind of food
- Body or talcum powders
- Body soap
- Carpeting
- Chlorine in water
- Clothing fabric
- Coffee
- Conditioner
- Deodorant
- Dishwashing soap
- Fingernail polish
- Hair mousse

(continued)

- Hair spray

- Household cleansers of all types

- Juice or milk

- Makeup

- Mattresses

- Medicinal creams or ointments

- Moisturizing lotion

- Mouthwash

- Perfume

- Pillows

- Shampoo

- Sheets and blankets

- Soft drinks

- Toothpaste

EXTERNAL ENVIRONMENT: INDIRECT CONTACT

- Bleach

- Fabric softener

- Heating or air conditioning systems

- Laundry detergent

- Paint

- Starch

- Wood stain

ENVIRONMENTAL TOXINS: ATMOSPHERIC

- Auto emissions

- Dust

- Industrial plant emissions

- Mold

- Pollen

- Wood smoke

The only way to deal with an excess of toxins is to determine what the toxin is and then remove it from your system. Sometimes this is easy, such as when your system is rejecting a food or a shampoo. Other times, it's more complicated. My daughter's situation is a good example. She has a chronic cough in the wintertime. When she was three years old, I was in the habit of spooning out the cough medicine every night before bed. It didn't seem to do much, but it made me feel as though I was at least attempting to help her.

One day, she swallowed an entire bottle of cough medicine. As we rushed her to the emergency room, she continued coughing. As she quite cheerfully cooperated with the emergency room staff, she was still coughing. I then realized that the medicine I was giving her did nothing at all except assuage my concern.

She survived the bottle of medicine without a glitch, but the cough persisted. I tried eliminating dairy from her diet. It made no difference. I put a humidifier in her room. Still no improvement. I tried plain logic: If the cough vanishes every summer, then we can rule out food, animal, pollen, grass, and other potential allergens. That wasn't much comfort. I finally resorted to pulling my hair out, but that did nothing except make me grumpy.

Eventually, I got smart and took her to Lee. He deduced that she has a sensitivity to our forced-air heating system. We cleaned out the ducts and pipes, but that didn't relieve the cough, either. Our only solution, then, was to move. Either that or wait it out. Unsure if we'd find a house with better or worse conditions, we stayed in our house and accepted that winters would be rough on our daughter's sensitive system. Not an easy choice.

More typically, however, eliminating a toxin is as simple as no longer ingesting something, changing the sheets, or switching to another brand of cleanser. Sometimes it means doing away with what you think is keeping you healthy. Too much exercise is a good example of this. So is taking medication.

Jake is in his seventies and was told by his doctor that he had glaucoma. He was on several different kinds of eyedrops to help with the condition. As time went on, his eyes began to produce a gluey substance that made it difficult for him to keep his eyes open. The doctor said to wait it out, and that it was probably a mild irritation of sorts. After several months, Jake reported that the situation was worsening. The doctor gave him more drops to help alleviate the irritation.

By the time Jake visited Lee, he could barely open his eyes. Lee's examination determined that Jake was allergic to the initial drops he had taken for the glaucoma. He took Jake off the medication, recommended another kind of drops to help with the glaucoma, and sent him home.

You know the end of this story. Within weeks, Jake's eyes were back to normal, and he continues to effectively treat his glaucoma with his new drops.

It doesn't matter if 40 percent of the people in a controlled study do well with a specific medication—if you're one of the 60 percent that doesn't, then you shouldn't take it. Negative side effects to medications can be an individual's allergic reaction to it. It doesn't do any good to take more medicine to clear up the reaction. If you're allergic, you need to stop imposing the substance on your system. Even if the allergic symptoms clear up with another medication, the sensitivity to the first one remains in your system, causing imbalances that can surface later as different symptoms. It's irrational to put a bandage on a wound if you're going to continue aggravating the wound from the other side of the skin.

Bill had a chronic dry cough for nine years before visiting Lee. He had been to four different medical doctors, and each one had conducted a battery of tests. Three of them admitted that they didn't know why Bill had the cough, but they assured him that it was no danger to his health. The fourth doctor said the cough was due to post-nasal drip. As a child, Bill had a lot of allergies and practically lived on nasal sprays. Consequently, as an adult, he has no sense of smell. Bill decided the fourth doctor was right, that he was just born with chronic post-nasal drip that irritated his throat and caused the cough.

Bill's belief changed after visiting Lee. According to the SOS Lee received from Bill's body, the cough had nothing to do with a congenital condition. It was, rather, an allergic reaction to coffee. Bill only drank two or three cups a day, but even so, his body simply didn't like it, which resulted in the persistent cough. When Bill quit drinking coffee, the cough was gone. Even though he still drinks it on occasion, he is relieved to know what causes his cough and how he can stop it once and for all, if he chooses.

Eliminating toxins from the body is usually easy, but it does take commitment. One woman I know has an extremely sensitive system, and consequently eats a very restricted diet. Her weakness, however, is diet soda. When she drinks it, her energy is depleted, but her commitment to stop hasn't kicked in. It's the one thing she indulges in and can't yet muster what it takes to stop. That's fairly common. We're all swayed by our culinary favorites. But the good news is that when she's ready, she'll know what to do to feel better and more energetic.

The Repertoire of Effective Treatments

There are many other treatment choices that can facilitate balance in your system. Lee has seen each one of the options discussed below work when they were introduced at the appropriate time. So, for example, if you have tried homeopathic remedies before and thought they were worthless, consider that they may not have been the appropriate answer to the problem you had at the time. But just because it didn't work before doesn't mean it won't work now. Again, ask the practitioner you work with to test your body to make sure it's responding favorably to the treatment of choice.

Herbs. TCM, Western herbs, or a combination of both are readily available and can be very useful. Take the list of Chinese herbs mentioned in "Generic versus Custom-Blended Herbs" on page 85 to your practitioner, and find out if these could work for your body. Capsule form and tinctures are both effective. Your TCM practitioner can also provide any number of immune-boosting herbs to stave off illness and keep you in the best possible shape for balancing the IBS.

Both singular and combination homeopathic remedies. We mentioned these in Chapter Two. If you muscle test well for homeopathic remedies, find a homeopathic or naturopathic doctor to treat you. There are hundreds of remedies, and it may be the best use of your time to work with a practitioner who is well versed in the choices and who can properly introduce them to your system.

Cell salts. Available in sugar tablets, these are beneficial for strengthening the very cells in your body—including those related to the digestive system.

Phyto-nutrients such as blue-green algae and wheat grass. These can help clean out the system.

Carotenoids, as typically found in beta-carotene. These rid your body of free radicals, which are another possible cause of imbalances.

Garlic. This comes in odor-free capsules, but the best kind is straight from the bulb. It's also a time-tested digestive aid.

Mushrooms. Shiitake, red reishi, and maitake are ancient remedies full of antioxidants that boost the immune system. If your health food store doesn't carry them, ask who might, or surf the Internet for sources.

Even if a certain treatment only works for 1 percent of the population, at least that 1 percent will finally be symptom free. Every option is worth mentioning and pursuing so that you can find the one that's right for you.

Emotional Components of Imbalance

As you can see, a wide range of different physical influences can cause IBS. Emotional energies or a combination of both physical and emotional upsets can also cause it. Even medical doctors acknowledge that stress is a trigger for some symptoms of IBS. Keep in mind that your physical body is denser than your refined emotional and spiritual bodies, but everything feeds into the pot of your overall health.

In some cases, it's difficult to know whether the original imbalance was due to an emotional or a physical cause. Your IBS could have started out as a physical problem, such as a thyroid deficiency. That, in turn, enervated you. Being tired all the time then made you grumpy and resentful of feeling bad, which in turn worsened the IBS. It's just as likely, however, that it happened in the opposite way. The initial cause could have been emotional in nature, rooted in feelings of unworthiness, for example. Then, in an attempt to prove yourself worthy, you burned the candle at both ends, which in turn created a thyroid deficiency. It simply doesn't matter how it first came about. Either way, in this situation, you need to deal with both a thyroid deficiency and your feelings of unworthiness. The goal is to restore a healthy balance, and to that end, it's important to acknowledge that chronic problems often have several different causes, and some of them may be emotional in nature.

Stress is a catchall phrase for a long list of aggravations. Discerning which emotional energies you throw into the brew of your overall well-being can help clear up the muddy waters of the imbalance. You may harbor deep resentment, trigger-happy anger, uncontrollable fear, or rampant worry—any number of heavy emotions. Any negative emotion can cause or contribute to IBS. When you understand which emotions or feelings have a hold on you, you can work to dissolve them and restore a healthy balance so it flows freely again.

Just like physical imbalances, emotional ones are typically due to an excess or deficiency. Earlier in the book, we mentioned a list of common reasons for stress due to excess, such as too much work, partying, answering to others' needs before your own, and so on. Deficiencies may include a lack of positive feelings toward yourself or others, but the primary deficiency in our culture and among most people is unencumbered time. You need this time in which you do nothing at all and you revel in that space.

> "If you can spend a perfectly useless afternoon in a perfectly useless manner, you have learned how to live."
>
> —Lin Yutany

Modern Roles, Stress, and IBS

We've already made it clear that we don't put much stock in statistics borne out of laboratory tests, but there is something to be said for statistics borne out of social trends. You may recall that more women than men reportedly have IBS. It's also true that more women than men are diagnosed with low thyroid. That's an interesting fact to know, given that low thyroid, according to Lee, is more often than not linked to people who are overachievers or workaholics.

In today's world, it's no wonder that women—especially working mothers—are on the go 24/7. But men, too, are fulfilling new roles in an attempt to balance their work lives with family activities. Finding a functional balance between meeting financial demands and fulfilling the unique needs of family members can take years to sort out. Even people *without* children are confronted with the stresses of rush hour, careers, being physically fit, and taking time for recreation. No matter what the situation, life in this day and age is fast-paced and requires a great deal of energy.

That said, life *can* be lived with reasonable balance. Everyone— no matter what design his life has taken on—must take responsibility for his own life story. If you resign yourself to the idea that life in the twenty-first century means you have to be stressed out, then you aren't honoring yourself. Instead, you're answering to impossible demands, trying to please others, or attempting to live up to an image you have of yourself that cannot reasonably be attained. This is the point at which your emotions will become unbalanced—or even unhinged—and after that, physical demise is just around the corner.

Stress is the nonphysical breakdown of the system by which you live. Who wouldn't break down after being on call twenty-four hours a day? It simply isn't possible to maintain good emotional or physical health with that lifestyle.

"If we only wanted to be happy, it would be easy; but we always want to be happier than other people, which is almost always difficult since we think them happier than they are."

—Ashley Montequie

Breaking the Cycle of Stress

Most people, regardless of gender, feel they have no choice but to go about their lives despite the madness of stress. They feel stuck. If that's true for you, then you have either stopped realizing, have forgotten, or have never learned that your life is where it is because you put it there. And it's up to you, and in your power, to change it.

Getting through life unscathed is a highly unusual feat. The prophets and masters can set the example, but most of us have to work pretty hard at it. As Lee says, "Life is the task at hand." Living it in physical and emotional balance is a choice that only you can make, and you must continue to make that choice on a daily basis. To thoroughly heal, you must take responsibility for this task and see it through to completion.

The most obvious step to releasing the stress in your life is to make different choices in your physical life so that you have more down-time. This may require that you finally break years of ingrained habits. Learn to say no. Delegate housecleaning chores to your spouse and children. Refuse to volunteer at the church bake sale. Ask someone else to pick up the kids at soccer practice. Let the house gather dust bunnies so you can put your feet up. Exercise, take a yoga class, learn how to meditate, sit on your front porch and watch the world go by. If you can't seem to force yourself to stop, enroll yourself in an art class or book club, or schedule a weekly or monthly massage. When you show up at the appointment or meeting, you will have no choice but to do something enjoyable and reenergizing.

Do not—absolutely and positively do not—turn on the television and call that sufficient downtime. And don't take a nap and call that your break. Watching TV and sleeping don't count. Do something every day, if possible, that stops your body from chasing down "have to's" and that nurtures your mind and spirit.

Making new physical choices is just the beginning; you also need to pay attention to the thoughts and images you house in your mind. The thoughts you think set the energetic tone for your body, as well as position your mental attitude. Start to notice how your thoughts make you feel. Do you think the world is good and safe, and so feel trusting of the process of life? Or do you think thoughts of doom and destruction and therefore are always awaiting disaster? Do you watch violent movies or TV shows that depict brutal murders and deranged people? If so, how do they make you feel about the world? About people? About the future of humankind? About walking out your front door? Ask yourself this: Could some of your IBS stem from violence you allow yourself to watch? Do you have flare-ups while watching the images? It's certainly worth noting.

Everything you put into your mind resonates with a specific energetic frequency. That frequency goes into the chemistry of your well-being. If you're addicted to horror films, then adrenaline will be part of your everyday mix, and sooner or later, it will probably manifest physically. If you surround yourself with music, poetry, and nature, you will absorb the energy of those forces, and they, too, will find a physical expression. If you operate on the premise that everything is energy, then be mindful that everything you say, read, watch, and participate in is going to influence—either positively or negatively—your emotional and physical health. The energetic nature of what you put into your mind and body is always your choice.

🌿

Monkey See, Monkey Do

A study led by Dr. B. J. Bushman of Iowa State University sought to define the relationship between media violence and aggression in children. Dr. Bushman's conclusions were published in a handbook released in 2001 titled "Effects of Televised Violence on Aggression." Here's an excerpt of what he found:

"True experiments have shown conclusively that exposing children to violent TV causes them to behave more aggressively immediately afterwards. Cross-sectional field studies have shown conclusively that the children who are watching more violence on TV are the same children who are behaving more aggressively. Longitudinal field studies have shown that children who grow up watching a lot of TV violence are likely to behave more aggressively later in childhood, in adolescence, and in young adulthood. This finding holds up even if one controls for differences in initial aggressiveness, intellectual functioning, and social class. The bottom line is that, on the average, TV violence is making our children behave more aggressively in childhood, and the aggressive habits they learn from TV in childhood carry over into adolescence and even young adulthood."

Start listening to yourself more closely, too. Do you choose words that accurately reflect what you really mean, or are you careless with your communication? If so, you may often feel misunderstood. Do you frequently yell at your loved ones? Does your boss yell at you? How do words, voices, and tone of voice affect you? Do you sense judgment in the tone of others? Are you aware of the judgment that may be in your tone? If thoughts were suddenly broadcast over loud-speakers and no one was able to conceal what they really think, would you be embarrassed most of the time? Proud? Confident? Mortified? What do you think you would learn about what other people think?

The answers to these questions provide subtle but very telling clues about what's going on in the emotional universe you and the people around you occupy. You may become aware that certain emotional energies take up more time and space in your mind than you'd like. You may begin to understand how they contribute to your symptoms. The first step in changing these thought patterns is to become aware of them. Then you can work at not allowing yourself to give them your time and attention.

Like most people, I've been prone to thinking fearful thoughts. Everything from the simple ones, such as "What if I encounter a wild animal on a hike?" to the most dramatic: "What if I'm in an earthquake and the house crumbles down and traps my children and I'm stuck beneath a huge beam and can't save them?" At some point along the way, I found myself obsessing on fearful thoughts. It was an addiction of sorts. I'd lie in bed unable to sleep as I felt a near-urgent need to cover all the worst-case scenarios I could conjure up in my mind. Inevitably, the more I focused on these thoughts, the faster my heart beat, the shorter my breath became, and the less chance I had of falling asleep. The sleepless nights rolled into sluggish days during which my brain didn't work very well, and a sliver of fear nipped at my heels throughout the day. It was a lousy way to go through life.

During that time, I visited Lee about a physical imbalance that was occurring. (Gee, I wonder why I had a physical problem during a time when *I could only think horrible thoughts!*) He dialogued with my body, did an acupuncture treatment, and put me on a flower essence. I had heard of flower remedies, but figured some hippie farmer who wanted to make a buck had created them back in the '60s.

I trusted Lee, however, and he assured me it would help with the emotional stuff that was going on inside me. Even though I didn't mention these obsessive thoughts to him, I later found out that the remedy he suggested for me was specific to breaking up the energy of fear and anxiety.

After taking the tincture for just a day, the shroud of fear lifted from me. Within two days, I was free of fearful thinking. It was then that I was able to look more objectively at my situation and myself and realize that I had *allowed* myself to become obsessive. Once I was free of the fear, I vowed not to let myself "go there" again.

Staying true to that promise required diligence and commitment. After all, it was an addiction of sorts. I came up with a phrase that speaks the truth to me and that keeps me from obsessing on the fearful thoughts. Whenever I notice such thoughts enter my mind, I speak that truth to myself, and it keeps me from giving in to the addiction. If I need extra support, I reach for the flower essence. Breaking stubborn and destructive thought patterns is another way to stop the cycle of stress.

> "There is only one way to happiness and that is to cease worrying about things which are beyond the power of our will."
>
> —Epictetus (50-120 A.D.)

Loosening the Energetic Pattern of Emotions

If you find it difficult to wean yourself from negative thoughts or images, Lee recommends approaching it from an energetic level. His tool of choice is exactly what he gave to me: flower remedies.

The energetic essence of certain flowers is highly refined, similar to emotional energy. When you take a flower remedy, you answer to the emotion at its own frequency. So, for example, when I experienced the obsessive and fearful thoughts in my mind, the remedy I took matched the energy within me and responded to it. The result was that it broke loose the energetic pattern I had created by allowing the thoughts to enter and take root in my mind.

Herbs can be effective for balancing upsets caused by biological dysfunctions. Two such examples are using St.-John's-wort to relieve mild depression and taking valerian for insomnia. But if the imbalance is generated primarily from an emotional source, even herbs are too dense to work out the kinks. That's when flower essence comes into play.

Rather than being created by a hippie looking for fame and fortune, flower remedies were created in the 1920s by a British medical doctor named Dr. Edward Bach. Dr. Bach had decided to dedicate his life to learning what causes illness, and according to the "Bach Flower Essence Guide to Personal Formulas," he believed that if a patient's emotional balance could be corrected, the body's natural ability to throw off illness would be strengthened automatically.

What ensued from Dr. Bach's studies was the development of thirty-eight remedies, all of which are available at health food stores. Homeopathically prepared from the flowers of nonpoisonous plants, bushes, and trees, each one targets specific mental and emotional states. When ingested, negative energies are apparently transformed into positive ones. There are no side effects and no contraindications with medications or other natural remedies.

Flower remedies, meditation, sitting in a rocking chair and watching the birds or squirrels—these are invaluable and important ways to spend time. In this highly yang world, allow the presence of yin in your life.

You now have a kit full of new and exciting tools. Use it. Take it to someone and get muscle tested for answers. This could be the beginning of your true recovery.

"Most people are about as happy as they've made up their minds to be."

—Abe Lincoln

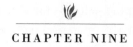

CHAPTER NINE

Maintaining Equilibrium: Habits for a Lifetime of Health

"By three methods we may learn wisdom:
First, by reflection, which is noblest;
Second, by imitation, which is easiest;
And third, by experience, which is bitterest."

— *Confucius*

When you first picked up this book, you may have thought you'd already done everything possible to treat your IBS, relieve the pain, and spend more time out of the bathroom than in it. However, now you're aware of many new options for treatment, including working with someone who may be able to articulate the very cause of the problem. This is powerful stuff. If you act on what you've learned here, you could find yourself living a different life than the one you've been acting out since you felt that first excruciating pain in your gut or realized that the diarrhea wasn't going away.

If you are truly committed to finding the cause of and solution to your IBS, we trust you will be successful in turning your life around. Even if you prefer not to work with an energy healer, a disciplined regimen of acupuncture and Chinese herbs will likely release you from years of discomfort and lead you down a healthier path. But once on the road to recovery, your next—and lifelong—charge is to maintain the good health you've searched so long and hard to find.

Learning to walk the line that separates balance from misery is an ongoing process. It can mean making significant lifestyle changes. It can require that you stay forever alert to the changing needs within you. As an upright and breathing chemistry lab, you'll probably find that what worked for you when you were twenty years old will not work for you when you're fifty. Heck, what worked for you last month may not work for you today. This shouldn't discourage you, however, because your toolbox is full. Over time, you will learn to recognize and interpret the signals your body sends out. Maintenance will become an adventure, and good health will become a way of life.

Our objective in writing this book was to fill your toolbox with the wisdom of the ancient healing arts of China, as well as with the latest discoveries in wellness. Staying true to that objective, we're now going to top off the toolbox with guidelines that are both old news and basic everyday knowledge. Namely, you have to eat well, exercise, and attend to your emotional, intellectual, and spiritual needs to maintain true health and balance. Body, mind, and spirit, remember? Even though this agenda sounds like a broken record, we promise to leave you with at least some new ways of carrying out that charge. So don't put down the book yet, assuming that you know what we're going to say. We've surprised you so far with strange new concepts, right? Well, we're not finished yet!

144 The IBS Breakthrough

"Quit worrying about your health. It'll go away."

—Robert Orben

Eating for Health and Vitality

So much media attention has been given to how and what we eat in America today that you'd have to be a hermit not to know some of the fundamental rules of eating well. Even so, we're going to review the party line for what's considered healthy, challenge a few of those tenets, and serve up a good portion of new ideas.

Here is what we're told to do to nourish our bodies and be wise eaters:

- Eat a healthy breakfast. Stay away from the eggs and bacon. Rather, eat low-fat cereals, jam on your toast, and fruit.
- Eat lean meats, only. Or even better, eat a salad instead of a burger.
- Choose mustard instead of mayonnaise.
- Avoid fast food joints.
- Eat less protein and more carbohydrates.
- Avoid fat whenever possible.
- Drink alcohol in moderation.
- Drink eight to ten glasses of water every day.
- Consume plenty of whole grains, fresh fruits, and vegetables.
- Supplement your diet with calcium and a good multivitamin.
- Fill up on fiber.

You'll notice the underlying message of these nutritional tips is to eat a low-fat diet. That makes sense, given the high incidence of obesity among American adults and the fact that 20 percent of our nation's children are overweight—and the percentage is rising. Seems reasonable enough, except for one crucial point. Our bodies require three ingredients to be healthy and function optimally: proteins, carbohydrates, and fat. Yes, fat. So what does this mean?

> "There is no sincerer love than the love of food."
> —George Bernard Shaw

You may already know that there are good fats and bad fats. You consume bad fats when you chow down on those greasy fast foods that are so darn satisfying—and so darn effective at widening your girth and clogging your arteries. Hydrogenated, partially hydrogenated, and saturated fats are those that increase your chances of heart disease and obesity. Unfortunately, these fats are found in a lot of great-tasting foods, including desserts, certain cuts of beef, chicken skin, and other yummy morsels. Finger-licking good or not, bad fats are truly the gangsters of the food chain, and they can kill off your chances of living a balanced and healthy life. Instead of simply avoiding fats, in your quest to be well you should avoid eating:

- All hydrogenated and partially hydrogenated oils
- Coconut oil
- Deep-fat-fried foods
- Lard
- Palm oil
- Processed foods (such as luncheon meats and smoked and cured meats like bacon, sausage, pepperoni, jerky, hot dogs, plus all premade or prepackaged foods)
- Saturated fats
- Shortening

Bad fats are even in some foods that you think are good for you, such as margarine and the low-fat versions of salad dressings, nondairy creamers, sandwich spreads, and other artificial foods.

The reason these foods are so hard on you is because the human body cannot process either bad fats or artificial foods. Processing or cooking these fats damages their structure and, as is true with artificial foods, our bodies don't recognize or know how to use them. And when the body cannot put the fats to use, they go to waste—on your waist, thighs, hips, belly, and even in your arteries. We're not entirely sure what happens with the artificial foods, but it's fairly typical to have some kind of subtle allergic reaction to them, such as headaches and muscle aches, but most likely digestive trouble.

Because fat has been largely responsible for heart disease and obesity, a huge movement ensued in America encouraging us to clean out the fat and eat lean. Sadly, the movement has thrown the baby out with the bath water. Instead of focusing on avoiding bad fats and ingesting good ones, there's a widespread belief that no fat is a good fat.

Here's a news flash for you: If you don't eat good fats, you will not become or stay healthy. Fat is crucial for certain biological functions that are necessary to have a healthy body. First, it plays a huge role in metabolism. Fat is what keeps it running at the perfect temperature and pace. Fat also transports the fat-soluble vitamins to their various destinations. It provides backup in times of famine (hey, you never know . . .), and it insulates our ever-important internal organs while also ensuring the production of sex hormones. So, although we may be the most overweight nation in the world, we could arguably be among the most undernourished because we don't eat enough of the right foods and good fats.

According to Lee, autoimmune deficiencies are responsible for the myriad chronic diseases that plague us these days, including fibromyalgia, multiple sclerosis, chronic fatigue syndrome, headaches, and so on. Through years of practice, he's determined that diet is the origin of many of these problems, and the biggest nutritional deficiency is good fat.

It's conceivable that your IBS may be caused by the lack of healthy fat in your diet. Lee gives an example of a teacher who experienced all the usual symptoms of irritable bowel syndrome. After the frustration of finding little relief from medical doctors, she asked Lee for help. Upon dialoguing with her body, Lee found that it was "screaming for fat."

🌿

Low Fat/No Fat = Low Health/No Health

"Are you fatigued? Not sleeping well? Do you have heartburn and other intestinal problems? Low-fat dieting promises health, but instead makes you unhealthy. Even if you are overweight, if you are eating a low-fat diet, you are starving your body. Every day that you eat a low-fat diet, your metabolism slows down. . . . No matter what else a person does, low-fat dieting dramatically compounds damage to his or her metabolism because virtually eliminating two essential nutrient groups (protein and fat) upsets the balance that the human body needs for constant nourishment. Low-fat dieting accelerates insulin resistance and aging, which leads to degenerative disease."

—Diana Schwarzbein, M.D.
The Schwarzbein Principle

Lee's answer to this deficiency and what he refers to as his "secret of all secrets" is extra virgin olive oil. He recommends that people with severe imbalances consume four to six tablespoons per day for one month. Those with a lesser dysfunction can get by on one or two tablespoons per day. He advises that everyone ingest one or two tablespoons per day just to ensure that there is enough good fat in everybody. You can take it in whatever way you like, including dribbling it over pasta, rice, or salad; dipping good bread into it; or cooking with it. Lee believes olive oil is just as important to our systems as essential fatty acids.

"If you don't have enough good fat in your body, everything breaks down," says Lee. "People are so fat-phobic these days that they're willing to risk their health just to be thin. Good health doesn't work that way."

If the idea of a tablespoon a day to keep the doctor away scares you off, bear in mind that Lee is not advising that you add olive oil to a diet already high in saturated or hydrogenated fat. First, eliminate the bad fats; then you can add the good fat with the confidence that it won't add excess weight. Many of Lee's patients have reported that upon making olive oil part of their daily routine, cravings for high-calorie sweets and carbohydrates have diminished.

"When your body gets the fat it needs, you're satisfied. You no longer need to nibble on foods high in bad fats when your overall need for fat has been satisfied."

Here's more good news, if you're concerned about gaining weight by taking this advice: Consuming olive oil may actually hasten weight loss. That's because if your body doesn't have enough good fat, your metabolism slows down. Shedding weight becomes a longer, more strenuous process. Lee says that by having a sufficient supply of good fat, your metabolism speeds up and enables you to lose weight in a healthier and more efficient manner.

"The first order of business is to get and be healthy," Lee reminds us. "Losing weight is usually a natural byproduct of having enough good fat in your system and eating the foods that work for you."

"I'm not a vegetarian because I love animals; I'm a vegetarian because I hate plants."

—A. Whitney Brown

Holly's Story, Age 49

I've had a problem with gas for about ten years. I don't know what kicked it in, but it's been the most embarrassing thing in my life. I've tried eliminating foods to see what caused it, but no matter what I ate or didn't eat, I'd go to bed each night with a distended stomach and painful gas.

When I went to Lee, he asked about the kinds of fat I eat. I told him I've been on a low-fat diet for the last ten years. After evaluating me, he said my body was short on good fat, and to take six tablespoons of olive oil every day. The thought of that was horrifying! I have a good body and I was terrified of gaining weight. But I was willing to try it because the gas was such a bother.

It's been four weeks now, and I haven't gained any weight. That's reassuring, but it's also understandable. Ever since I started with the olive oil, I've lost my desire for meat and sugar. I used to have at least one sweet a day, but now I just don't want it. It's not that I've quit eating meat, but before the olive oil, I used to feel the need to eat it. Now I don't, so I'm eating lighter: more vegetables, fish, and rice, and no dessert. The best news of all is that this new way of eating has reduced the gas. I still have my moments, but for the most part, it's far less painful and it doesn't happen nearly as much.

Recognizing Appropriate and Inappropriate Foods

Finding the foods that work for you can also be a process. I don't do well digesting bananas. In all my years of writing about health, I've never read that bananas might be hard on the system. But the truth is, they're hard on mine. You, too, have a unique system that will respond favorably to some foods and unfavorably to others. Even foods considered good and necessary by most experts may not ultimately work for your system.

You may find, for example, that all those good, whole-grain foods exacerbate your IBS. The key may be that you are sensitive to gluten, an ingredient in wheat-based whole-grain products. Typical allergic reactions to gluten include all the regular IBS symptoms: abdominal cramping, distended stomach, gas, and irregular bowels. Work with your practitioner to determine which foods to avoid, or keep close track of what happens to you after you eat, and respond accordingly.

Consider, too, that a combination of different foods can affect how you feel and can cause symptoms to flare up. Some people cannot digest protein and starches in the same meal. Others can, but if they finish their meal with fruit, they end up paying. Each digestive system has its own unique chemistry, and it's up to you to learn what works for you and what doesn't. Bookstores are full of resources on food combining. If you suspect your system becomes sensitive only when you eat certain foods at the same sitting, there are plenty of ways to learn more about it.

> "To eat is human
> To digest divine."
> —Mark Twain

Lee illustrates the need to respect individual needs by telling the story of Randy, a beef-eating Texan in his late sixties. Randy came to Lee carrying nearly one hundred extra pounds, having no energy, and riddled with aches and pains. To make matters worse, his medical doctor told Randy that he only had a few years left to live. Not because of cancer or another fatal disease, but because his internal organs weren't functioning well. He was wearing out.

After examining Randy, Lee put him on a pituitary supplement, told him to stop eating all animal products, and had him start taking six tablespoons of olive oil each day. Randy's wife was a nutritionist and balked at the idea of eliminating animal products—and olive oil, of all things? Even so, Randy felt that he had no choice but to try it.

Two months later, Randy visited Lee with twenty fewer pounds, a big grin, and renewed energy. Even some Texans don't do well eating red meat.

As a general rule, Lee suggests reducing intake of animal protein (including dairy products), sugar, coffee, red wine, and hard alcohol. He advises completely eliminating artificial sweeteners.

As the years go by, your body will change and so will its tolerance for some foods. Be receptive to your body's needs during the cycles of your life. Vitality is an awesome payoff.

Exercise: The Elixir for Elation

Whether you're a veteran couch potato and have absolutely no interest in exercise or you're an expert on endorphins, the simple truth is that maintaining health requires regular exercise.

"Health nuts are going to feel stupid someday, lying in hospitals dying of nothing."

—Redd Foxx

There are tens of thousands of resources explaining the benefits of and the best ways to exercise. We're not going to gloss over a subject that is so important to your health and so eloquently detailed in all those books, videos, and classes. Rather, we're simply here to remind you that refusing to exercise is, in a way, choosing to stagnate the Qi within you. By now, you know that stagnant Qi leads to both physical and emotional imbalance.

If the idea of jumping around in a gym, pounding across miles of running trails, and biking up steep grades doesn't appeal to you, consider pursuing one of the martial arts. If you like the basic philosophy of TCM, you can extend your knowledge and incorporate it into your daily physical routine. Qigong (chee-gong), tai chi, aikido, karate, and other martial arts combine exercise with meditation. Since they are precise movements tied in with specific intentions that can have a profound affect on your health, it's best to learn them from a qualified teacher. Ask your TCM practitioner for guidance. He or she may actually teach the classes, since certain disciplines, such as qigong, are

🌿

Movement as a Meditation on Health

"In order to maintain health, you have to have physical movement, but also meditative balance. And you have to control not only your physical body, but also your will and intention and your thoughts. Without that mental overlay, the physical movements are just superficial calisthenics. In traditional Chinese medicine, you don't just do calisthenics to get your heart rate up, and you can't just sit and meditate all day. One without the other is not enough. The combination is at the heart of Chinese medicine."

—Dr. David Eisenberg
in Bill Moyers's *Healing and the Mind*

very much a part of the culture of Chinese healing. Visit bookstores or the Internet to find out more about the martial arts.

Whatever you choose to do for exercise, do it knowing that it will become one of the most important aspects of your life. It will sustain you through difficult times and will nourish your body, mind, and spirit.

Spiritual Significance

"Nothing can bring you peace, but yourself."

—Ralph Waldo Emerson

Your toolbox brimming with useful instruments, but what good is it, regardless of how full it is, if you can't unlock it? According to TCM, your health and spiritual life are a continuum, uninterrupted by space or time. It's all energy, remember? That means that if you neglect your spiritual life, you may lose—or never find—the key to your toolbox.

Studies show that people who practice some kind of religious or spiritual faith live longer and heal faster than those who don't. It doesn't matter which faith they participate in; what matters is that they believe there is an order larger than their lives, or their own understanding, within each moment and event. Perhaps because of this, they are more accepting, and so more at peace with whatever unfolds.

Spiritual or religious practice is based on a very personal choice and subjective experience. Unfortunately, politics has penetrated most branches of it, which may be why some people shy away from it. But everyone is tugged by the same questions: Why am I here? What is my purpose? What difference does my life make in the big picture? How can there be a God when there is so much evil and sickness in the world?

There is no single answer to any one of these questions, but if you don't sit with them and seek your own meaning, you'll be left with no answers at all. Healing yourself and being whole are one and the same. Developing a spiritual life is as important as eating well, exercising, and giving and receiving love.

Rather than bid you farewell and good luck on your journey to health by closing with borrowed wisdom from Chinese sages, we'll leave you with a passage that could spark innate wisdom of your own:

". . . the spiritual test inherent in all our lives is the challenge to discover what motivates us to make the choices we do, and whether we have faith in our fears or the Divine. We all need to address these questions as a matter of spiritual thought or as a result of physical illness. We all reach a moment when we ask, Who is in charge of my life? Why aren't things working out the way I want? No matter how successful we are, at some point we will become conscious that we feel incomplete. . . . Gaining an awareness of our own limitations opens us to considering choices we would not otherwise have made. During moments when our lives seem most out of control, we may become receptive to guidance that we would not have welcomed before. . . . It may help you to arrive at the point of surrendering if you can use symbolic sight to view your life as only a spiritual journey. We have all known people who have recovered from dire circumstances—and credited the fact that they let the Divine take over. And every one of these people shared the experience of saying to the Divine, 'Not my will but Yours.' If that one prayer is all that is required, why are we so afraid of it?"

—Caroline Myss
Anatomy of the Spirit

RESOURCES

Adderly, Brenda, ed. *The Complete Guide to Pills*. New York: Ballantine Books, 1996.

Bushman, B. J., and L. R. Huesmann. "Effects of Televised Violence on Aggression." *Handbook of Children and the Media* by Dorothy G. Singer and Jerome L. Singer. Thousand Oaks, California: Sage Publications, 2001.

Cassidy, Claire, Ph.D. "Chinese Medicine Users in the United States: Part I: Utilization, Satisfaction, Medical Plurality." *The Journal of Alternative and Complementary Medicine, Volume 4, Number 1*, 1998, pp. 17–27.

Cassidy, Claire, Ph.D. "Chinese Medicine Users in the United States, Part II: Preferred Aspects of Care." *The Journal of Alternative and Complementary Medicine, Volume 4, Number 2*, 1998, pp. 189–202.

Chopra, Deepak. *Namaste* online newsletter

Giuffre, Kenneth, M.D. *The Care and Feeding of Your Brain: How Diet and Environment Affect What You Think and Feel*. Franklin Lakes, NJ: Career Press, 1999.

Gomi, Taro. *Everyone Poops*. Brooklyn, NY: Kane/Miller Book Publishers, 1993.

Moore, Thomas J. *Prescription for Disaster: The Hidden Dangers in Your Medicine Cabinet*. New York: Dell, 1999.

Moyers, Bill. *Healing and the Mind*. New York: Doubleday, 1993.

Myss, Caroline, Ph.D. *Anatomy of the Spirit: The Seven Stages of Power and Healing*. New York: Harmony Books, 1996.

Schwarzbein, Diana, M.D., and Nancy Deville. *The Schwarzbein Principle: The Truth about Losing Weight, Being Healthy, and Feeling Younger.* Deerfield Beach, FL: Health Communications, 1999.

Tolle, Eckhart. *The Power of Now: A Guide to Spiritual Enlightenment.* Novato, CA: New World Library, 1999.

Wilhelm, Richard, and Cary F. Bynes, trans. *The I Ching, or Book of Changes.* Princeton, NJ: Princeton University Press, 1967.